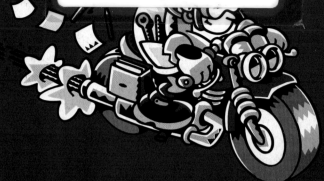

Renal and Urinary Systems

Series editor
Daniel Horton–Szar
BSc (Hons)
United Medical and Dental
Schools of Guy's and
St Thomas's Hospitals
(UMDS),
London

Faculty advisor
Kevin PG Harris
MA, MD, FRCP
Senior Lecturer/Honorary
Consultant Nephrologist
University of Leicester
School of Medicine and
Leicester General Hospital

Renal and Urinary Systems

Nisha Mirpuri
BSc (Hons)
United Medical and Dental
Schools of Guy's and
St Thomas's Hospitals
(UMDS),
London

Pratiksha Patel
United Medical and Dental
Schools of Guy's and
St Thomas's Hospitals
(UMDS),
London

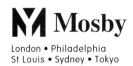 Mosby

London • Philadelphia
St Louis • Sydney • Tokyo

Editor	Louise Crowe
Development Editor	Filipa Maia
Project Manager	Nigel Wetters
Designer	Greg Smith
Layout	Gisli Thor
Illustration Management	Mike Saiz
Illustrators	Sandie Hill
	Jenni Miller
	Marion Tasker
	David Graham
	Robin Dean
	Amanda Williams
	Debra Woodward
Cover Design	Greg Smith
Production	Gudrun Hughes
Index	Janine Ross

ISBN 0 7234 3126 4

Published by Mosby, an imprint of Harcourt Publishers Limited, Robert Stevenson House, 1-3 Baxter's Place, Leith Walk, Edinburgh EH1 3AF, UK.

Printed in Barcelona, Spain, by Grafos S.A. Arte sobre papel.
Text set in Crash Course–VAG Light; captions in Crash Course–VAG Thin.

The publisher, author and faculty advisor have undertaken reasonable endeavours to check drugs, dosages, adverse effects and contraindications in this book. We recommend that the reader should always check the manufacturer's instructions and information in the British National Formulary (BNF) or similar publication before administering any drug.

Cataloguing in Publication Data
Catalogue records for this book are available from the British Library.

As the medical curricula have evolved, the scientific basis and clinical aspects of each speciality have become increasingly integrated. *Crash Course Renal and Urinary Systems* reflects today's curricula by integrating the basic science with clinical topics. In this book, we have tried to explain topics in the way we understand them, from the student's perspective.

The information has been set out in a way that is easy to read and learn from. Numerous diagrams and algorithms have been used to simplify some of the more complex principles. We have used hints and tips boxes where we needed to highlight important points and comprehension check boxes help you to check your knowledge as you go along.

The structure of the book follows the renal and urinary systems from basic anatomy and physiology through to history taking, physical examination, and pathology.

We both found the renal and urinary systems to be a very challenging aspect of our course and hope that *Crash Course Renal and Urinary Systems* will provide a complete and simplified review for your learning.

Good luck in your exams!

Nisha Mirpuri
Pratiksha Patel

The primary aim of *Crash Course Renal and Urinary Systems* is to provide the medical student with a framework of knowledge for the study of these systems. The text is designed with the new medical curriculum in mind and interlinks basic science with clinical medicine.

As with the other books in the *Crash Course* series, this book for medical students has been written by medical students with expert input from the Series Editor and myself as the Faculty Advisor. This innovative approach has ensured that the text is user friendly, easy to follow, and accurate.

In using a concise text with extensive illustrations, the emphasis has been to produce a balanced book covering renal physiology and pathophysiology in a way that will give the student a solid overview of the subject. At the same time, the theoretical basis relevant to the problems they will encounter in everyday clinical practice has been provided. Unnecessary complexity has been avoided without loss of relevant practical information.

It is hoped that this book will provide students with a useful supplement to their lecture notes, stimulate them to continue with self-directed learning in this subject, and provide them with a concise yet comprehensive revision aid. To this end a comprehensive set of multiple-choice questions, short-answer questions, and essay topics, together with answers, are provided for the reader to test his or her knowledge.

Any suggestions or criticisms from readers which would help us better attain these objectives in the future would be greatly appreciated.

Kevin Harris
Faculty Advisor

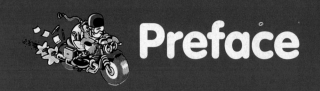

Preface

OK, no-one ever said medicine was going to be easy, but there are very few parts of this enormous subject that are actually difficult to understand. The problem for most of us is the sheer volume of information that must be absorbed before each round of exams. It's not fun when time is getting short and you realise that: a) you really should have done a bit more work by now; and b) there are large gaps in your lecture notes that you meant to copy up but never quite got round to.

This series has been designed and written by medical students and young doctors with recent experience of basic medical science exams. We've brought together all the information you need into compact, manageable volumes that integrate basic science with clinical skills. There is a consistent structure and layout across the series, and every title is checked for accuracy by senior faculty members from medical schools across the UK. I hope this book makes things a little easier!

Danny Horton-Szar
Series Editor

Acknowledgements

Thanks to Danny, Dr Harris, Nigel, and everyone at Mosby for putting in a great amount of time and effort in bringing this book together. It's been hard work, but a very enjoyable and valuable experience. We would also like to thank our families and friends who have supported us and put up with all our moaning over the past year.

Figure Credits

Figures 2.5 and 2.30 taken from Human Histology 2e, by Dr A Stevens and Professor J Lowe. TMIP. 1997.

Figures 2.16 and 4.1 taken from Integrated Pharmacology, by Professor C Page, Dr M Curtis, Professor M Sutter, Professor M Walker, and Professor B Hoffman. Mosby, 1997.

To our parents, Bhabi, Bejul, Sameer, and Shalini

for their love, inspiration, and support.

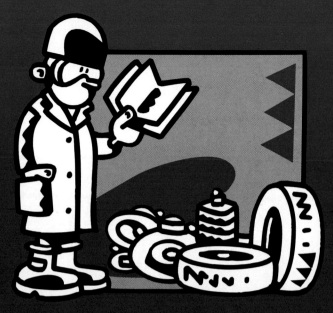

DEVELOPMENT, STRUCTURE, AND FUNCTION

OVERVIEW OF THE KIDNEY AND URINARY TRACT

Functions of the kidney

The kidneys are the major organs responsible for maintaining at a constant level the composition and volume of the body fluids—homeostasis.

They have several functions, which can be summarized as:

- Regulation of water content, mineral composition, and acidity of the body by excreting substances in an amount adequate to achieve total body balance and maintain normal concentration in the extracellular fluid.
- Elimination of metabolic waste products from the blood and their excretion in urine (e.g. urea from protein metabolism, uric acid from nucleic acids, creatinine from muscle creatine).
- Removal of foreign chemicals from the blood and their excretion in urine (e.g. drugs, pesticides, food additives).
- Secretion of hormones (endocrine function)—erythropoietin (controls erythrocyte production), renin (generates angiotensin I from angiotensinogen and controls blood pressure and sodium balance), 1α hydroxylase enzyme (metabolism of vitamin D), and prostaglandins (vasodilator effect).

Embryology of the kidney and the urinary tract

Three consecutive systems form the adult urinary tract:

- Pronephros, which develops in the cervical region of the embryo and is rudimentary.
- Mesonephros, which has characteristic excretory units with their own collecting ducts called mesonephric ducts or wolffian ducts. It develops in the thoracic and lumbar regions as the pronephros regresses. It may function for a short time.
- Metanephros (permanent kidney), which develops at about week 5 in the pelvic region. It forms excretory units (nephrons) from the metanephric mesoderm, and the collecting system is formed from the ureteric bud, which is an outgrowth of the mesonephric duct.

The metanephric tissue forms a cap over the ureteric bud, which grows and divides to form the renal pelvis, calyces, and collecting ducts.

The connection between the collecting system and the nephrons is essential to the normal development of the urinary tract. Any failure in this process may cause unilateral or bilateral renal agenesis. Cystic disease can also result from failure of development of the ureteric bud or the kidney tissue. Early division of the ureteric bud results in bifid kidneys, occasionally with ectopic ureters. Abnormal migration of the kidneys into the abdomen from their original position in the pelvis results in pelvic or horseshoe kidneys (see Chapter 9).

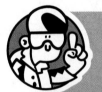

Understanding that the kidneys develop in the pelvic region and migrate into the abdominal cavity will help you understand anomalies such as pelvic kidneys.

Structure of the kidneys and urinary tract

The kidneys are located retroperitoneally on the posterior abdominal wall and lie either side of the vertebral column. The right kidney is 12 mm lower than the left (because of displacement by the liver). A kidney measures approximately 11 cm long, 6 cm wide, and 4 cm thick.

Each kidney is composed of about 1 000 000 nephrons bound together by small amounts of connective tissue containing blood vessels, nerves, and lymphatics. Each nephron consists of:

- Glomerulus, which forms a protein-free and cell-free filtrate of blood.
- Tubule, which processes the filtrate as it flows through the tubule before exiting the kidneys as urine.

Fig. 1.1 shows the anatomy of the kidneys and urinary tract.

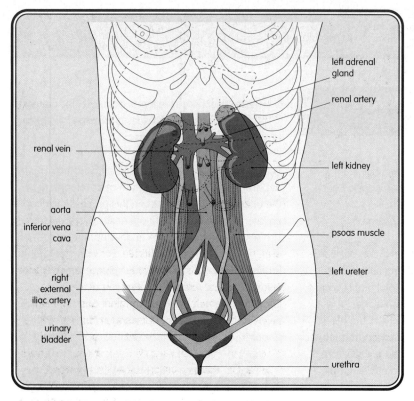

Fig. 1.1 Anatomy of the posterior abdominal wall showing the kidneys and urinary tract.

left adrenal gland

renal artery

renal vein

left kidney

aorta

inferior vena cava

psoas muscle

right external iliac artery

left ureter

urinary bladder

urethra

- What are the functions of the kidneys?
- Give a brief description of the location and structure of the kidneys.
- What are the three stages of embryological development?

FLUID COMPARTMENTS OF THE BODY

Body fluids

Body fluids are divided into:
- Intracellular fluid (ICF), the fluid within cells.
- Extracellular fluid (ECF).

ECF is divided into:
- Plasma—ECF within the vascular system.
- Interstitial fluid (ISF)—ECF outside the vascular system (and separated from plasma by the capillary endothelium).
- Transcellular fluid (TCF)—ECF (e.g. synovial fluid, aqueous and vitreous humour, cerebrospinal fluid) (Fig. 1.2) separated from the plasma by the capillary

endothelium and an additional epithelial layer that has specialized functions.

Water is a major component of the human body. Approximately 63% of an adult male and 52% of an adult female is water (i.e. 45 L in a 70 kg male, 36 L in a 70 kg female). One-third of total body water (TBW) is ECF (about 15 L in a 70 kg male) and two-thirds is ICF (about 30 L in a 70 kg male).

Osmolarity and osmolality
Basic concepts

Osmosis is the net passage of a solvent through a semi-permeable membrane between two solutions of different strengths until equilibrium is reached. The osmotic effect can be measured as an osmotic

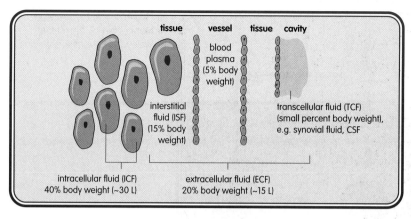

Fig. 1.2 Fluid compartments of the body.

tissue   vessel   tissue   cavity

blood plasma (5% body weight)

interstitial fluid (ISF) (15% body weight)

transcellular fluid (TCF) (small percent body weight), e.g. synovial fluid, CSF

intracellular fluid (ICF) 40% body weight (~30 L)

extracellular fluid (ECF) 20% body weight (~15 L)

pressure. Hydrostatic pressure is the pressure needed to be applied to the region containing the solute to prevent the net entry of water.

The total solute concentration of a solution is known as its osmolarity—the number of osmotically active particles in solution. The higher the osmolarity, the lower the water concentration. 1 Osm = 1 mole of solute particles.

Osmolarity vs osmolality

Osmolarity is the molar concentration per litre of solution (mOsm/L). Osmolality is the molar concentration of solutes per unit weight of the solvent (water) (mOsm/kg H_2O).

- Normal body fluid osmolality is 280–290 mOsm/kg H_2O.
- Urine osmolality can vary in the range 60–1400 mOsm/kg H_2O.

Plasma osmolality can be calculated from Na, K, urea, and glucose concentrations with the formula:

Plasma osmolality = 2(Na + K) + urea + glucose

Isotonicity and isosmoticity

Changes in the extracellular osmolarity can cause cells to shrink or swell as water will move across the plasma membrane by osmosis out of or into the cells. Therefore a major function of the kidneys is to regulate the excretion of water in the urine so that the osmolarity of the ECF remains nearly constant despite wide variations in intake or extrarenal losses of salt and water. This prevents damage to the cells from excess swelling and shrinkage:

- If cells are placed in a solution of 300 mOsm/kg H_2O (isotonic solution, i.e. 0.9% saline), there is no net movement of water by osmosis and no swelling or shrinkage.
- If cells are placed in a solution of less than 300 mOsm (hypotonic solution), they swell as water osmoses into the cell.
- If cells are placed in a solution of over 300 mOsm (hypertonic solution), they shrink as water moves out of the cell.

Fig. 1.3 shows the changes in the cells brought about by hypertonic, isotonic, and hypotonic solutions.

Isosmoticity refers to the osmolarity of a solution relative to that of cells regardless of whether the solutes are penetrating or non-penetrating. Isotonicity refers to the osmolarity of a solution relative to its non-penetrating solutes regardless of its concentration of membrane-penetrating solutes (e.g. 300 mOsm/L of non-penetrating solutes).

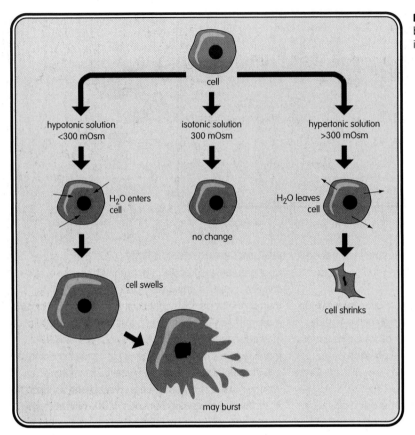

Fig. 1.3 Changes in the cells brought about by hypertonic, isotonic, and hypotonic solutions.

Diffusion of ions across biological membranes

Biological membranes (e.g. cell membranes) are selective in that they allow diffusion of small molecules and ions through them. The concentration gradient and electrical gradient are important in the movement of these molecules.

Diffusion of different molecules occurs at different rates depending upon their shape, size, weight, and charge.

When solutions either side of a membrane contain only freely diffusible ions, the electrical gradient causes ions to move from an area of high ionic concentration to one of low ionic concentration until equilibrium is reached and the ion distribution will be such that the products of the concentration of diffusible ions of the two sides will be equal as follows:

Side A (diffusible cations × diffusible anions) =
Side B (diffusible cations × diffusible anions)

When non-diffusible anionic protein is present on one

Sodium (Na^+) is the main extracellular ion. Potassium (K^+) is the main intracellular ion.

side of the membrane, cations will cross the membrane to maintain electrical neutrality. This will cause the side containing non-diffusible ions (e.g. protein) to have a slightly greater number of total ions than the side containing only diffusible ions; therefore the osmotic pressure on the side with the non-diffusible ions will be greater. Net water movement will then occur unless the osmotic pressure difference is counterbalanced by hydrostatic pressure.

Cell membranes are permeable to:
- Potassium ions (K^+).
- Chloride ions (Cl^-).
- Sodium ions (Na^+).

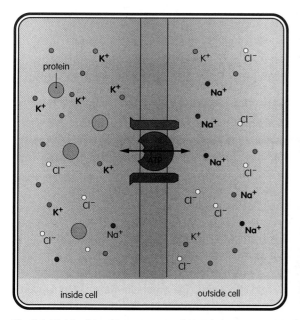

Fig. 1.4 Distribution of ions across cell membranes.

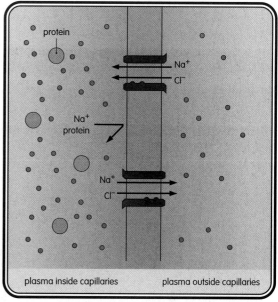

Fig. 1.5 Influence of protein on diffusible ions across cell membrane—demonstrating the Gibbs–Donnan effect.

The permeability of Na^+ is 1/50th of K^+ permeability. The primary active transport mechanism uses adenosine triphosphate (ATP) actively to pump Na^+ out of and K^+ into the cells, but most K^+ in the cell is present as a result of high permeability. Cl^- ions diffuse out of the cell across the cell membrane because there is a net negative charge within the cell. This results in a higher concentration of Cl^- ions outside the cells. At equilibrium, the cell has a net negative charge (−70 mV). Fig. 1.4 shows the distribution of ions on either side of the cell membrane.

Proteins (large molecules):
- Are almost impermeable to the membrane.
- Are mostly anionic and influence the diffusion of other ions, thus causing an imbalance in the distribution of diffusible ions—the Gibbs–Donnan effect (Fig. 1.5).

According to the Gibbs–Donnan effect, there should be more ions inside the cell than outside. These are, however, balanced in biological systems by the sodium pump as Na^+ is effectively non-diffusible.

Fluid movement between body compartments

Body fluid compartments have a relatively constant yet dynamic composition. Equilibrium is maintained by the continual transfer of fluid between the different compartments.

Exchange between ECF and ICF

Water freely diffuses across cell membranes so that equilibrium is reached between the ICF and ECF. Any change in the ionic concentration of the ICF or ECF is followed by the movement of water between these compartments. Na^+ is the most important extracellular osmotically active ion. K^+ is the most important intracellular osmotically active ion.

Exchange between plasma and interstitial fluid

The capillary endothelium separates plasma from interstitial fluid (ISF). Water and ions move between these two compartments, 90% of ions by simple diffusion and 10% by filtration.

Ion filtration between plasma and ISF is carried out through:
- The arterial end of the capillary where there is a hydrostatic pressure of 32 mmHg, which causes fluid to filter out of the plasma into the ISF.
- Proteins that are too large to cross the capillary endothelial cells and therefore remain in the plasma, creating a colloid osmotic (or oncotic) pressure (25 mmHg).
- The venous end of the capillary where there is an osmotic pressure of 25 mmHg, which is greater than the hydrostatic pressure (12 mmHg). This causes fluid to return to the capillary.

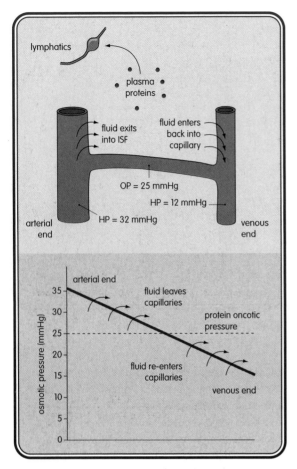

Fig. 1.6 Exchange of fluid between the plasma and ISF across a capillary wall. (HP, hydrostatic pressure; OP, oncotic pressure.)

Composition of fluid compartments			
Component	Plasma	ECF	ICF*
Na^+ (mmol/L)	142	145	12
K^+ (mmol/L)	4	4.1	150
Cl^- (mmol/L)	103	113	4
HCO_3^- (mmol/L)	25	27	12
proteins (g/L)	60	0	25
osmolality (mOsm/kg H_2O)	280	280	280
compartment volume (L)	3.0	12.0	30

*ICF compartment is not the same throughout the body; it varies with different types of cells

Fig. 1.7 Composition of the fluid compartments.

The exchange of fluid between the plasma and ISF across a capillary wall is illustrated in Fig. 1.6. Hydrostatic pressure depends upon arteriole blood pressure, arteriole resistance (which determines the extent to which blood pressure is transferred to the capillary), and venous pressure.

Osmotic pressure (25 mmHg) is produced by plasma proteins (17 mmHg—oncotic pressure) and the imbalance of ions—there are more ions (e.g. Na^+) inside the capillary than outside as a result of the presence of negatively charged proteins and the Gibbs–Donnan effect.

Exchange between interstitial fluid and lymphatic vessels

Some plasma proteins can be lost from the vascular system into the ISF. The lymphatic system is composed of a network of lymphatic capillaries in all organs and tissues, which eventually join to drain into the venous system via the thoracic duct in the neck. These lymphatic capillaries are very permeable to protein and thus return the escaped plasma proteins to the circulatory system.

The ionic composition of the fluid compartments is shown in Fig. 1.7.

Fluid and ion movement between the body and external environment

There is a continuous exchange of body fluids with the external environment, but there must be a balance between intake and output.

Water intake and output are illustrated in Fig. 1.8. Water lost from the lungs varies with the climate (e.g. in very dry climates over 400 mL per day is lost). Insensible losses are those due to evaporation of water from the skin (i.e. not sweat). Sweating ('sensible perspiration') is an additional loss. Urinary loss can be varied according to the needs of the body. Intakes also vary considerably and can be adjusted according to need (i.e. thirst mechanism). Despite these variations, the body's ionic concentration is maintained within strict limits by the kidney mechanisms, including control of tubular reabsorption of filtered Na^+ and to a lesser extent K^+.

Water intake and output			
Water intake (mL)		**Water output (mL)**	
drink	1500	lungs	400
food	500	skin	400
metabolism	400	faeces	100
		urine	1500
total	2400	total	2400

Fig. 1.8 Water intake and output.

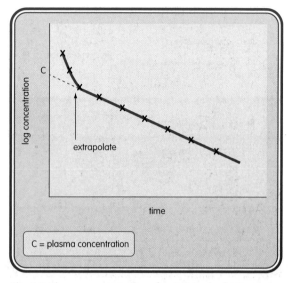

C = plasma concentration

Fig. 1.9 Plasma concentration of an injected substance.

Measuring body fluid compartments
Dilution principle

The dilution principle is used to measure fluid volume when fluids cannot be directly measured or extracted from the container or compartment holding them. This allows measuring *in situ*. A substance that will mix completely and uniformly in the fluid compartment is used to allow all of the volume present to be measured. Allowances must be made for the excretion and metabolism of substances by the body.

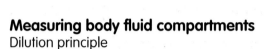

$$V_D = \frac{Q_A - Q_H}{C}$$

Where V_D = volume of distribution; Q_A = quantity administered; Q_H = quantity metabolized after 10 hours; C = concentration.

   Two methods are used:
- Single injection method.
- Constant infusion method.

Single injection method

This is used when the substance has a slow rate of excretion from the compartment being measured and is carried out as follows:
1. A known amount of test substance is injected intravenously.
2. Plasma concentration is determined at intervals.
3. A graph (log concentration against time scale) is plotted (Fig. 1.9).
4. Extrapolate the straight portion to time 0—this gives the concentration of substance that will distribute evenly instantly (Fig. 1.9).

Using this method:

$$\text{Compartment volume} = \frac{\text{Amount injected}}{\text{Concentration at zero time}}$$

Constant infusion method

This is used for test substances that are rapidly excreted and is carried out as follows:
1. A loading dose of the test substance is injected intravenously.
2. The test substance is infused at a rate to match renal excretion rate.
3. Plasma concentration is measured at intervals.
4. When the substance comes to equilibrium, the plasma concentration is constant (Fig. 1.10).
5. Stop the infusion.
6. Collect urine until all the test substance has been excreted.

Using this method:

   Amount excreted = Amount present in the body at the time the infusion was stopped

And:

$$\text{Compartment volume} = \frac{\text{Amount excreted (mg)}}{\text{Plasma concentration (mg/L)}}$$

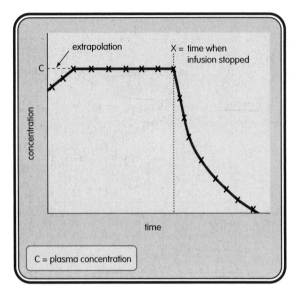

Fig. 1.10 Plasma concentration of an infused substance. (From Principles of Renal Physiology by C Lote, 1993.)

reinjecting, and determining the dilution of the label after 15 min.

Measurement of extracellular fluid

As ECF is made up of several compartments, it is difficult to measure accurately. A substance that will diffuse across the endothelial barriers into the ISF, but not into the cells, is required. It is difficult to measure the TCF as it is separated from the capillaries by another membrane in addition to the capillary membrane. Substances used include:

- Inulin (may be excluded from bone and cartilage).
- Mannitol.
- Thiosulphate (most widely used).
- Radiosulphate.
- Thiocyanate.
- Radiochloride or radiosodium (these substances cannot be completely excluded from cells).

Normal ECF volume = 15 L

Measurement of plasma volume, red cell volume, and blood volume

Plasma volume, red cell volume, and blood volume are measured as follows:

- Plasma volume—the test substance needs to remain within the vascular system (e.g. plasma protein) and radio-iodinated human serum albumin or Evans Blue dye are used.

  Normal plasma volume = 3 L

- Blood volume—measure the haematocrit (% of red blood cells in total blood volume) by centrifuging a small sample of blood—for example, if the haematocrit is 45%, the plasma volume is 55% of blood volume (measure plasma volume as above and blood volume = plasma volume × 100/55).

  Normal blood volume = 5 L

- Red cell volume can be measured from plasma volume and haematocrit or by direct dilution, which is carried out by taking a small sample of blood, incubating red blood cells in radioactive phosphorus (^{32}P) or chromium (^{51}Cr), resuspending (in saline),

Measurement of interstitial fluid

ISF cannot be measured directly. It needs to be calculated as follows:

ECF (15 L) − plasma volume (3 L) = ISF (12 L)

Measurement of total body water

Isotopes of water are used as markers (deuterium oxide or tritiated water) to measure total body water (TBW). A normal value in a 70 kg man is 63% (i.e. 45 L) and in a 70 kg woman, 52% (36 L), being lower in women because of their greater proportion of body fat.

Measurement of transcellular fluid

As this compartment is separated from the rest of the ECF by a membrane, the substances used to measure the ECF do not cross into this compartment. Thus TCF is included in the TBW, but excluded from the ECF, thus:

TBW = ECF + ICF + TCF

There is a large turnover—about 20 L/day for the gastrointestinal tract.

- What are the different fluid compartments of the body and what are their relative proportions and values?
- Define osmolality and osmolarity and give their units of measurement. What is normal plasma osmolality?
- What is the ionic composition of the different body fluid compartments?
- Describe how both ions and fluid move between the external environment and the body.
- How do we measure plasma volume, red cell volume, blood volume, ECF, ISF, TBW, and TCF?

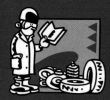

2. Organization of the Kidney

GENERAL ORGANIZATION OF THE KIDNEY

Macroscopic organization

The anatomy of the kidneys is shown in Fig. 2.1. Relationships of other organs to the kidneys are as follows:

- Anterior (Fig. 2.2)—to right kidney: liver, 2nd part of the duodenum, and the colon; to left kidney: stomach, pancreas, spleen, jejunum, and descending colon.
- Posterior—diaphragm, quadratus lumborum, psoas, 12th rib, and three nerves (subcostal, iliohypogastric, and ilio-inguinal).
- Medial—hilum (a deep fissure containing the renal vessels and nerves and the renal pelvis); to left kidney: aorta; to right kidney: inferior vena cava.
- Superior—adrenal gland.

The kidneys lie in an abundant fatty cushion (perinephric fat) contained within the renal fascia. They have three capsular layers:

- Fascial (renal fascia).
- Fatty (perinephric fascia).
- True (fibrous capsule).

Morphology and internal structure

Within the kidney, the ureter continues as the renal pelvis, which lies in a deep fissure called the hilum. The outer border of the renal pelvis divides into two or three major divisions (calyces), which in turn subdivide into a number of minor calyces. Each minor calyx is indented by a papilla of renal tissue called the renal pyramid, and it is here that the collecting tubules empty the urine. Along with the renal pelvis, the renal artery, vein, nerve, and lymphatics all enter the medial border of the kidney at the hilum (Fig. 2.3).

The kidney is divided into two main layers:
- Outer renal cortex.
- Inner renal medulla.

The glomeruli in the cortex give it a granular appearance on histology.

The blood supply of the kidneys is from the right and left renal arteries, which branch directly off the abdominal aorta at the level of L1–2. The renal veins drain the kidneys directly into the vena cava. Lymphatics drain to the para-aortic lymph nodes.

Nephrons

There are about 1 000 000 nephrons in each kidney.

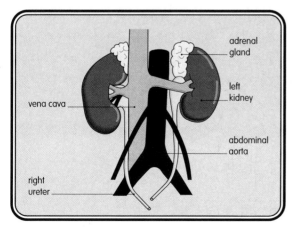

Fig. 2.1 Anatomy of the kidneys.

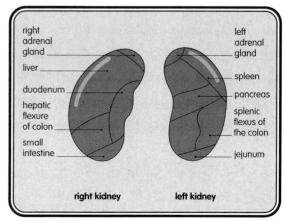

Fig. 2.2 Anterior relations of the kidney.

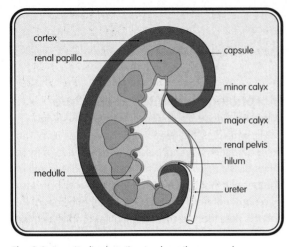

Fig. 2.3 Longitudinal section to show the general organization of the kidney.

The nephron is the functional unit of the kidney and consists of:
- A renal corpuscle (Bowman's capsule and the glomerulus).
- Tubule (proximal tubule, loop of Henle, distal tubule and collecting duct) (Fig. 2.4).

There are two types of nephron depending upon the length of the loop of Henle.
1. Nephrons with renal corpuscles in the outer part of the cortex that have corresponding short loops of Henle (cortical nephrons).
2. Nephrons in the inner third of the cortex with long loops of Henle extending down into the medulla (juxtamedullary nephrons).

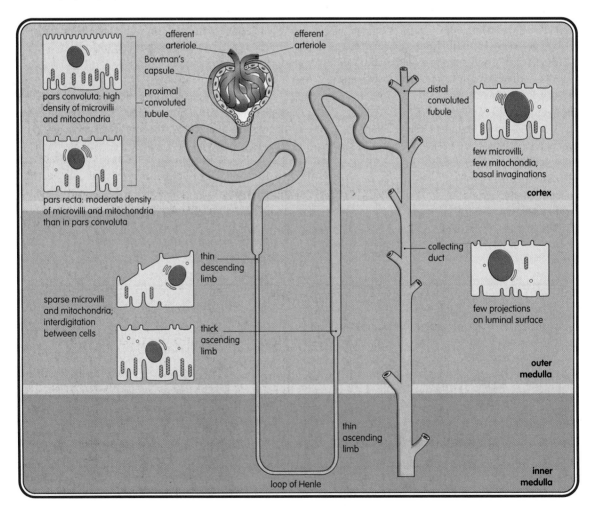

Fig. 2.4 Diagram to show the structure of a nephron and the main histological features of different cell types within the nephron.

Glomerulus

The glomerulus is formed by the invagination of a tuft of capillaries into the dilated blind end of a nephron (Bowman's capsule). It measures approximately 200 μm in diameter.

The function of the glomerulus is to produce a protein-free filtrate from the blood in the glomerular capillaries. The capillaries are supplied by the afferent arterioles and drained by the efferent arterioles. The filtration membrane of the renal corpuscle is made up of three layers and is fundamental to kidney function.

Proximal tubule

The proximal tubule continues from the renal corpuscle. It is 15 mm long and 55 μm in diameter. The wall is made up of a single layer of cuboidal cells, which interdigitate extensively with each other and are connected by tight junctions at their luminal surfaces. The luminal edge of each cell is made up of millions of microvilli, forming a dense brush border which provides a much greater surface area for absorption of tubular filtrate. At the base of each cell there are infoldings of the cell membrane (Fig. 2.4). Lateral extension of the extracellular space at the side of the cells is the lateral intercellular space.

The proximal tubule varies along its length:

- The first part is convoluted (pars convoluta) and cells have an increased density of microvilli and a greater number of mitochondria than cells in the second straight part, suggesting increased development of transport functions.
- The second straight part (pars recta) leads on to the first part of the loop of Henle (the thin descending limb).

Loop of Henle

The loop of Henle consists of a single layer of flattened squamous cells, which form a thin-walled hairpin-shaped tube.

The cells of the thin descending segment interdigitate sparingly with each other and have few mitochondria and microvilli on the luminal surface (Fig. 2.4). This segment ends at the tip of the hairpin loop.

The thin ascending segment has a 20 μm diameter and is 2 mm long. It has a structure that is similar to the preceding part of the tubule except that the cells have extensive interdigitations between them and functionally this may relate to active transport and permeability properties of the cells. There is an abrupt transition between the thin and thick ascending segments and the level of this depends upon the length of the loop.

The thick ascending segment is 12 mm in length and consists of a single layer of columnar cells. The luminal membrane is invaginated to form many projections, though there is no brush border and there are few infoldings of the basal membrane.

Distal tubule

The distal convoluted tubule is an anatomical term, describing the continuation of the loop of Henle into the cortex and ending in the collecting ducts. The cells have very few microvilli, no brush border, and basal infoldings surrounding mitochondria that gradually decrease towards the collecting ducts (Fig. 2.4). The basal membranes of all cells have Na^+/K^+ ATPase pump activity.

There are different cell types in this part of the tubule including:

- Principal cells (P cells), which are responsive to antidiuretic hormone (ADH)—also known as vasopressin.
- Intercalated cells (I cells), which secrete H^+.

Collecting ducts

The cortical collecting ducts are 20 mm long. They are lined with cuboidal cells that have a few projections on the luminal surface (Fig. 2.4). The ducts pass through the renal cortex and medulla, and at the apices of the renal pyramids drain the urine into the renal pelvis. The renal pelvis is lined by transitional epithelium.

In the cortex each collecting duct drains approximately six distal tubules. In the medulla the distal tubules join together in pairs to form ducts of Bellini and from here drain into the renal calyx.

Blood supply and vascular structure

The kidneys receive 20–25% of the total cardiac output (1.2 L/min). The blood enters the kidney via the right and left renal arteries. These branch to form about five interlobar arteries, which divide to form the arcuate arteries (these are located at the junction between the cortex and medulla). The interlobular arteries arise at 90 degrees to the arcuate arteries through the cortex, dividing up to form the afferent arterioles, which supply the glomerular capillaries.

The efferent arterioles drain blood from the glomerular capillaries, acting as portal vessels (i.e. carrying blood from one capillary network to another). In the outer two-thirds of the cortex the efferent arterioles form a network of peritubular capillaries that supplies all cortical parts of the nephron. In the inner third of the cortex the capillaries go on to follow a hairpin course adjacent to the loops of Henle and the collecting ducts down into the medulla. These vessels are known as the vasa recta. The vasa recta and the peritubular capillaries drain into the left and right renal veins and then into the inferior vena cava. The microcirculation of the kidney is illustrated in Fig. 2.5.

Function of the renal blood supply

The high rate of blood flow through the kidney is very important in maintaining the homoeostatic functions of the kidney. The blood flow through the kidney determines the filtration rate and 50% of the oxygen consumption is required for Na^+ reabsorption in the tubules. The oxygen consumption of the kidney is 18 mL/min.

Although there is a very large flow of blood, the arteriovenous oxygen difference is only about 15 mL/L compared with 62 mL/L in the brain and 114 mL/L in the heart (i.e. the oxygen extraction is not as efficient as in other organs as a result of shunting of blood in the vasa recta because of its hairpin structure).

Juxtaglomerular apparatus (JGA)

The JGA (Fig. 2.6) is located where the thick ascending loop of Henle passes back up into the cortex and lies adjacent to the renal corpuscle and arterioles of its own nephron. The association of the arterioles and the distal tubule is the area known as the JGA. The tunica media in the wall of the afferent arteriole contains an area of specialized thickened cells (granular cells), which secrete renin. The epithelium of the distal tubule is modified in this region to form a specialized type of cell (macula densa cells) that responds to the composition of the tubular fluid, especially the Na^+ concentration of the filtrate.

Renin acts on angiotensinogen to form angiotensin I, which in turn is converted to angiotensin II. Angiotensin II is a potent vasoconstrictor affecting blood pressure,
tubular reabsorption of Na^+, and aldosterone secretion from the adrenal glands. Stimuli for renin release include sympathetic stimulation of the granular cells or a decrease in filtrate Na^+ concentration. The latter may occur following a fall in plasma volume, vasodilation of the afferent arterioles, and renal ischaemia.

Contractile cells identical to the mesangial cells are found just outside the glomerulus in association with the glomerular apparatus—these are extraglomerular mesangial cells (Goormaghtigh cells) or lacis cells.

Erythropoietin (EPO)

The kidney is the major source (85%) of EPO production in the adult. In fetal life the liver also produces EPO. It is produced by the peritubular interstium and cells of the inner cortex. EPO-sensitive cells are the erythrocyte stem cells found in the bone marrow and the effect of the hormone is to increase the production of erythrocytes resulting in an increase in the oxygen-carrying capacity of the blood. The half-life of EPO is 5 hours.

Clinical use of erythropoietin

Hypoxia, anaemia, and renal ischaemia all stimulate EPO synthesis. Increased secretion is seen in polycystic kidney disease and renal cell carcinoma resulting in polycythaemia. Patients with chronic renal failure often have inappropriately low EPO secretion resulting in normochromic normocytic anaemia. Recombinant human EPO is used in patients with chronic renal failure.

Vitamin D

Vitamin D is obtained in the diet and is synthesized in the skin from 7-dehydrocholesterol in the presence of sunlight. This naturally occurring vitamin D (cholecalciferol) is hydroxylated in the liver to form 25-hydroxycholecalciferol [25(OH)D$_3$]. The second hydroxylation of 25(OH)D$_3$ occurs in the tubular cells of the kidney under the influence of the enzyme 1α-hydroxylase to form the biologically active metabolite 1,25-dihydroxycholecalciferol [1,25(OH)$_2$D$_3$]. The production of 1,25(OH)$_2$D$_3$ is regulated by parathyroid hormone (PTH), phosphate, and by negative feedback. Active vitamin D is essential for the mineralization of bones and plays an important role in calcium metabolism.

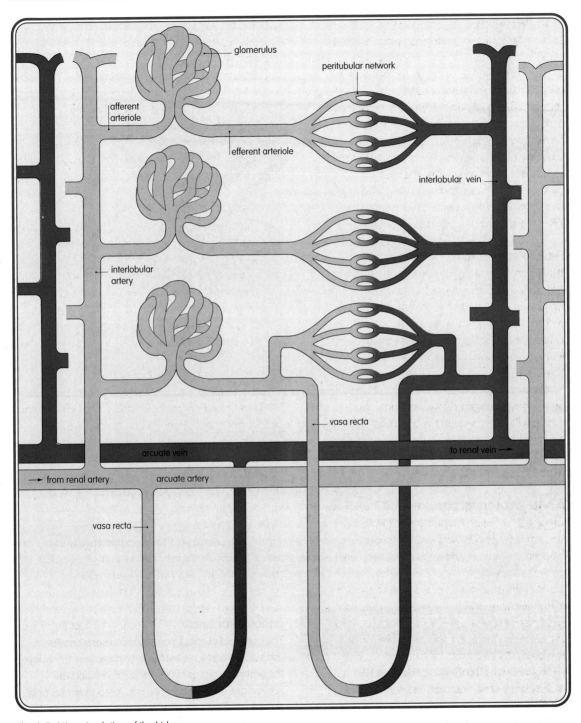

Fig. 2.5 Microcirculation of the kidney.

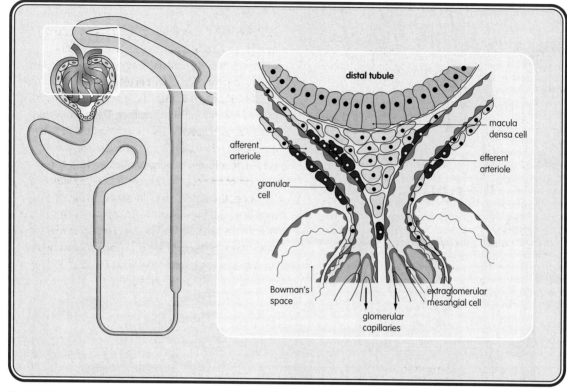

Fig. 2.6 Juxtaglomerular apparatus.

GLOMERULAR STRUCTURE AND FUNCTION

Structure of the glomerular filter

The first stage of urine production is the filtration of plasma through the glomerular capillary wall into Bowman's capsule. The composition of the ultrafiltrate of plasma is dependent upon the three layers of the filtration barrier (Fig. 2.7):

- The endothelial cells of the glomerular capillary.
- A basement membrane.
- The epithelial cells of Bowman's capsule.

Endothelial cells

The endothelial cells lining the glomerular capillaries are perforated by numerous fenestrae (pores), allowing the plasma components to cross the vessel wall. The pores have a diameter of 60 nm. The endothelial cells are thin and flat with a large nuclei. This layer of the filter prevents the filtration of blood cells and platelets.

Basement membrane

The basement membrane is a continuous layer of connective tissue and glycoproteins. It is a non-cellular structure and prevents any large molecules from being filtered.

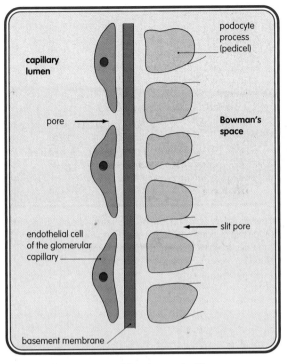

Fig. 2.7 Microstructure of the glomerular filter.

Epithelial lining

The epithelial lining of Bowman's capsule consists of a single layer of cells, which rest on the basement membrane and are called podocytes. The podocytes have large extensions or trabeculae, which project out from the cell body and are embedded in the basement membrane surrounding a capillary. There are small processes called pedicels, which extend out from the trabeculae and interdigitate extensively with the pedicels of adjacent trabeculae. This leads to the formation of slit pores, which control the movement of substances through the final layer of the filter. The podocytes have well-developed Golgi apparatus and a major function of these cells is the production and maintenance of the glomerular basement membrane. They may also be involved in phagocytosis of macromolecules (Figs 2.8 and 2.9).

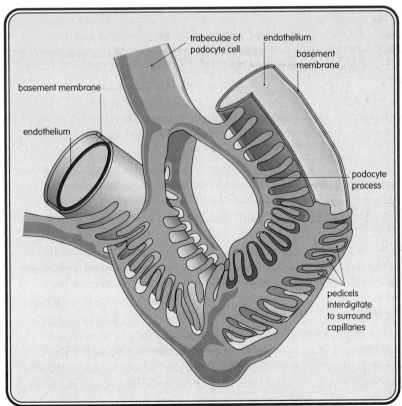

Fig. 2.8 Arrangement of the podocytes and pedicels.

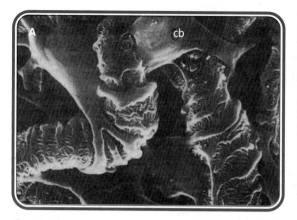
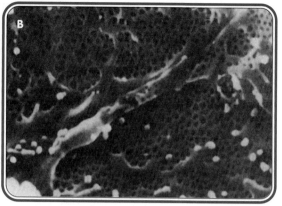

Fig. 2.9 Electron micrographs to show the arrangement of podocytes and glomerular capillaries as they would be seen from Bowman's capsule. (A) Processes of podocytes run from the cell body (cb) towards the capillaries where they ultimately split into foot processes (pedicels) . (B) Inner surface of a glomerular capillary. (From Renal Physiology, 2nd Edition. BM Koeppen, B Stanton. Mosby Year Book, 1996.)

To visualize the filter, imagine the glomerular capillaries being pressed into a very soft and stretchy balloon (the Bowman's capsule). In this way the entire surface of the capillaries will be in contact with the balloon.

Mesangium

The mesangium is also part of the of the renal corpuscle and consists of two components:
- Mesangial cells.
- Mesangial matrix.

The mesangial cells surround the glomerular capillaries and have a function similar to monocytes. They provide structural support for the capillaries, exhibit phagocytic activity, secrete extracellular matrix, and secrete prostaglandins. The cells are contractile, and this may contribute to regulation of blood flow though the glomerular capillaries (Fig. 2.10).

Process of glomerular filtration

The filtration of all macromolecules depends upon their molecular weight, shape, and charge. Filtration is a passive process and involves the flow of a solvent through a filter; any molecules that are small enough to pass through the filter form the filtrate. The glomerular filter allows only the low molecular weight molecules of the plasma to pass through it. These then make up the glomerular ultrafiltrate

Glomerular filtration rate (GFR)

The GFR is the amount of filtrate that is produced from the blood flowing through the glomerulus per unit time.
- Normal GFR is 125 mL/min/1.73m^2 (i.e calculated for body surface area).
- The total amount filtered is 180 L/day.

The glomerular filtrate normally:
- Is free of blood cells and platelets.
- Contains virtually no protein.
- Is mostly made up of organic solutes with a low molecular weight and inorganic ions.

Molecular size

Molecular weight is the main factor in determining whether a substance is filtered or remains in the capillaries. The molecular weight cut-off of the filter is 70 kDa. With macromolecules the shape of the molecule as well as its electrochemical charge affect filterability. All three layers of the filter are coated with anions and these repel negatively charged macromolecules like albumin. Smaller and positively charged molecules pass through the filtration barriers relatively easily, the only exception being any molecule bound to protein.

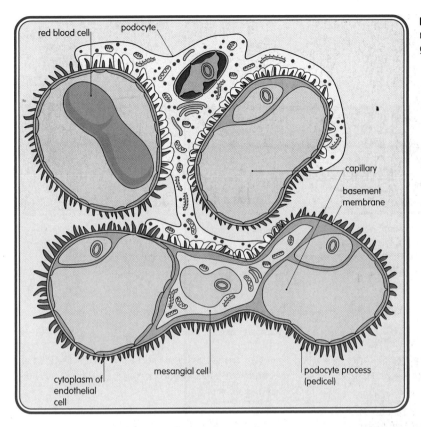

Fig. 2.10 Relationship between mesangial cells and the glomerular capillaries.

Labels: red blood cell, podocyte, capillary, basement membrane, podocyte process (pedicel), mesangial cell, cytoplasm of endothelial cell

Any molecule with a molecular weight of less than 70 kDa is freely permeable through the filter (e.g. glucose, amino acids, Na$^+$, urea, K$^+$).

Forces governing tissue fluid formation

The movement of fluid between the plasma and tissue fluid is determined by:

- Hydrostatic pressure.
- Colloid osmotic (oncotic) pressure (due to protein).

These are known as Starling's forces (Fig. 2.11).

Tissue fluid formation depends upon the following factors:

- At the arteriole end of the capillary hydrostatic pressure is much greater than colloid oncotic pressure as a result of resistance to flow due to the narrowing of the vessel, and fluid is forced out of the capillary—point 1 in Fig. 2.11A.
- As the fluid moves out of capillaries via the highly permeable wall the oncotic pressure increases and the pressure forces are reversed (most apparent at the venous end of the capillary) and there is net movement of fluid back into the capillaries—point 2 in Fig. 2.11A.

Forces governing GFR

In the renal vascular bed the surface area of the glomerular capillaries is much larger than that of normal capillary beds and therefore there is less resistance to flow. The hydrostatic pressure falls less along the length of the capillary because of the efferent arterioles, which act as secondary resistance vessels and so maintain a fairly constant pressure along the entire length of the glomerular capillary—point 3 in Fig. 2.11B.

The equivalent of tissue fluid in a vascular bed is the glomerular filtrate in Bowman's space, produced because of the hydrostatic pressure in the glomerular capillary (50 mmHg). The pressure in the glomerular capillaries is opposed by the hydrostatic pressure in Bowman's capsule (12 mmHg) and the colloid oncotic pressure (25 mmHg) within the capillary. When these forces are equal the filtration equilibrium is reached and there is very little fluid movement after this.

The fluid is reabsorbed into the peritubular capillaries—point 4 in Fig. 2.11B—as a result of the very high colloid oncotic pressure (35 mmHg) and very low hydrostatic pressure. This reabsorption results in a reduced colloid oncotic pressure as plasma proteins become diluted.

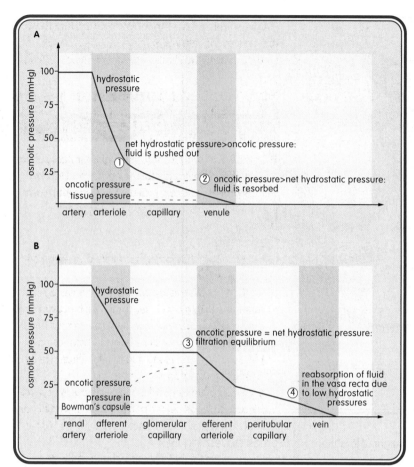

Fig. 2.11 Forces involved in tissue fluid formation in a non-renal (A) and a renal (B) vascular bed (numbers on the graphs correspond to the textual description on p. 21).

The pressures controlling glomerular filtration into Bowman's capsule are illustrated in Fig. 2.12 and the composition of the glomerular filtrate is shown in Fig. 2.13.

Albumin has a molecular weight of 69 000 and is negatively charged. Very tiny amounts get through the filter due to the repelling effect of its negative charge and all of this is reabsorbed in the proximal tubule. A total of 30 g of protein a day enters the renal lymph vessels. Significant amounts of protein in the urine are indicative of disease or infection in the urinary tract.

Feedback control of glomerular filtration
Tubuloglomerular feedback mechanism
The GFR remains constant over a wide range of arterial pressures. Because the flow through the capillaries governs the GFR, there must be a method of autoregulation within the renal circulation. The mechanism controlling this process is the tubuloglomerular feedback mechanism in which the composition of the distal tubular fluid can control the GFR for that nephron. The system requires three components:

- A luminal component that recognizes a certain parameter within the tubular fluid. The macula densa cells of the tubular epithelium detect osmolality or the rate of Na^+ or Cl^- movement into the cells. The higher the flow of the filtrate the higher the Na^+ concentration in the cells.
- A signal, which is then sent via the juxtaglomerular cells, as a result of any change in the NaCl concentration of distal tubular fluid.
- An effector (adenosine), which acts as a vasoconstrictor to contract the smooth muscle of the adjacent afferent arterioles and therefore decreases renal plasma flow, which in turn reduces GFR.

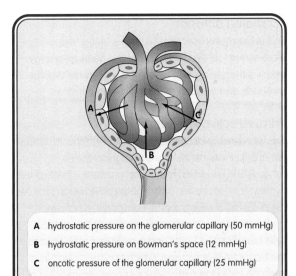

A   hydrostatic pressure on the glomerular capillary (50 mmHg)

B   hydrostatic pressure on Bowman's space (12 mmHg)

C   oncotic pressure of the glomerular capillary (25 mmHg)

Fig. 2.12 Pressures controlling glomerular filtration into Bowman's capsule.

Composition of glomerular filtrate	
Component	**Glomerular filtrate**
Na$^+$ (mmol/L)	142
K$^+$ (mmol/L)	4.0
Cl$^-$ (mmol/L)	113
HCO$_3^-$ (mmol/L)	28–30
glucose (mmol/L)	5.9
protein (g/100 mL)	0.02

Fig. 2.13 Composition of glomerular filtrate.

∘ **Describe the structure of the glomerular filter.**

∘ **How does the molecular size of particles affect filtration?**

This mechanism serves to maintain a constant GFR and prevents overloading of the nephron since a high NaCl load decreases the filtration capacity of that nephron.

TRANSPORT PROCESSES IN THE RENAL TUBULE

The ultrafiltrate produced from the glomerular filter has a composition similar to plasma and is modified by various processes (reabsorption and secretion) within the tubule to produce the final urine (Fig. 2.14).

Definitions

Definitions for reabsorption, secretion, and excretion are as follows:

- Reabsorption is the removal of substances from the tubular fluid into or between the cells lining the tubule, which then pass back into the circulation.
- Secretion is the process by which substances are removed from the blood into tubular filtrate via cells or intercellular spaces.
- Excretion is the removal of waste products from the blood and is the net result of filtration, secretion, and reabsorption of a substance.

Fig. 2.14 illustrates the processes that occur in the nephron and result in excretion of a substance. There are two types of transport of solutes involved in these processes:

- Paracellular movement (between cells) across the tight junctions that connect the cells where the driving forces are concentration and electrical and osmotic gradients.
- Transcellular movement (through cells) via both the apical and basal membranes and the cell cytoplasm where there is no active process for water absorption, but it follows the movement of solutes by osmosis.

Transport mechanisms
Diffusion

Diffusion is the simple movement of substances down their electrochemical gradient. It does not require any metabolic energy or carrier molecules and therefore the movement is passive.

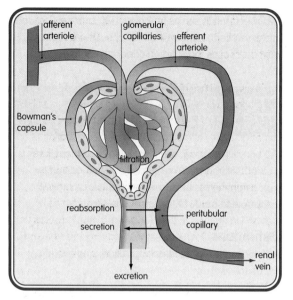

Fig. 2.14 Processes that occur in the nephron and result in excretion of a substance.

Facilitated diffusion

This is the movement of substances along their electrochemical gradient without the need for energy and it is therefore passive, but it does require a carrier molecule and is much more rapid than diffusion.

Primary active transport

This is an energy-dependent process in which substances are able to cross cell membranes against their concentration and electrochemical gradient. It involves the hydrolysis of adenosine triphosphate (ATP), which provides direct chemical energy for the transport mechanism.

The most important active process in the tubular cells found on the basal and basolateral membranes is the Na^+/K^+ ATPase pump, which transports Na^+ from intracellular to the extracellular spaces maintaining a low Na^+ concentration and a high K^+ concentration in the cells (Fig. 2.15). This pump allows the nephron to reabsorb over 99% of the filtered Na^+.

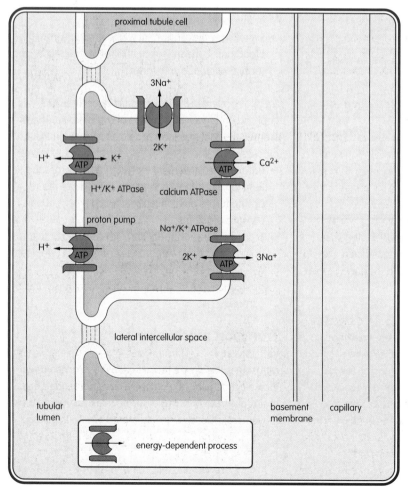

Fig. 2.15 Primary active transporters in the tubule cells:
- H^+/K^+ ATPase
- proton pump
- Ca^{2+} ATPase
- Na^+/K^+ ATPase (sodium pump).

The other primary active transporters on the tubular cell membrane are:

- Ca$^+$ ATPase.
- H$^+$/K$^+$ ATPase.
- H$^+$ ATPase.

The ATP molecule is an intrinsic part of the protein structure in the primary active transporters. The energy is derived from the hydrolysis of the terminal phosphate bond of the ATP molecule to form adenosine diphosphate (ADP) (Fig. 2.16).

Secondary active transport

This process uses the energy produced from another process for transporting molecules (i.e. the transport of the solutes is coupled). The most important example of this mechanism involves the Na$^+$/ K$^+$ ATPase pump as the driving force for the secretion and reabsorption of other solutes in which the energy is provided by the Na$^+$ gradient.

The Na$^+$/K$^+$ ATPase pump creates an ionic gradient across the cell membrane and this then allows the energy produced from diffusion of Na$^+$ into the cell as it moves along its electrochemical gradient to be used for the uphill transport (i.e. against their electrochemical gradient) of other solutes.

Substances can move in two directions by the following processes:

- Symport—energy produced by the movement of Na$^+$ is used to transport other substances in the same direction across the cell membrane (i.e. with the Na$^+$ gradient) (e.g. the Na$^+$/K$^+$/Cl$^-$ co-transporter in the thick ascending limb and the Na$^+$/glucose in the cells of the proximal tubule cells).
- Antiport—movement of substances against their electrochemical gradient in the opposite direction to the Na$^+$ gradient (e.g. the Ca^{2+}/Na$^+$ and the H$^+$/Na$^+$ exchangers).

These processes are carried out by carrier molecules that are specific protein structures in the cell membrane called transporters.

Ion channels

These are protein pores found on the epithelial cell membranes. They allow for the rapid transport of ions into the cell. There are Na$^+$, K$^+$, and Cl$^-$ specific channels on the apical membrane of all the cells lining the nephron. Although transport in these channels is very fast

(10^6–10^8ions/s) there are only about 100 channels per cell compared to the slower (100ions/s), but more numerous active transporters (10^7 transporters per cell).

Handling of sodium by the kidney

Using sodium ions (Na$^+$) as an example we can see how the filtrate is modified by various aspects of the nephron to produce the excreted product. The concentration of Na$^+$ in Bowman's capsule is equal to the plasma level since Na$^+$ is freely filtered. Virtually all the Na$^+$ that is filtered into the nephron is reabsorbed back into the circulation and only 1% or less of the filtered Na$^+$ is excreted in the urine. This is a very important process not only to preserve Na$^+$ levels in the body, but also because the reabsorption processes of glucose, amino acids,

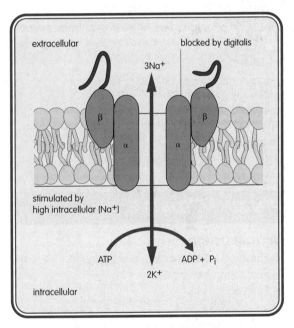

Fig. 2.16 Na$^+$/K$^+$ATPase pump found in the basal membrane of the cells. It drives secondary active transport by maintaining a low Na$^+$ concentration in the cells.

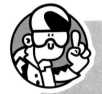

Generating Na$^+$ gradients within the kidney is central to the reabsorption of many substances, including glucose, amino acids, water, lactate, Cl$^-$, HCO$_3^-$, and PO$_4^{3-}$.

Na+ transport along the nephron			
Part of nephron	Percentage of filtered Na+ reabsorbed	Method of entry into the cell	Regulatory hormones
proximal tubule	65–70	Na+ co-transport, paracellular	angiotensin II
loop of Henle	20–25	Na+/Cl−/K+ pump (1:2:1)	aldosterone
early distal tubule	5	Na+/Cl− symport	aldosterone
late distal tubule and collecting ducts	5	Na+ channels	aldosterone, atrial natriuretic peptide

Fig. 2.17 Na+ transport along the nephron.

- Define reabsorption, secretion, and excretion.
- What is the difference between primary and secondary active transport?

water, lactate, Cl−, HCO_3^-, and PO_4^{3-} ions depend upon the movement of Na+ back into the cells of the tubule. Na+ transport along the nephron is shown in Fig. 2.17.

PROXIMAL TUBULE

Microstructure

The proximal tubule is made up of two parts:
- Pars convoluta.
- Pars recta.

The most active transport occurs in the cells of the pars convoluta. The features of a proximal tubule cell are shown in Fig. 2.18. Histology is discussed earlier (see Fig. 2.4).

Transport of sodium and chloride

Extrusion of sodium into the lateral space
70% of the filtered Na+ is reabsorbed in the proximal tubule. The primary transporter Na+/K+ ATPase (Na+ pump) on the basolateral membrane transports Na+ actively out of the cell into the lateral intercellular spaces between adjacent cells.

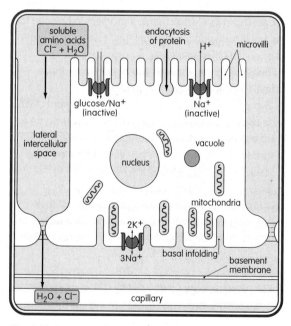

Fig. 2.18 Features of a proximal tubule cell.

Sodium entry into the cell

This movement of Na+ out of the cell maintains a very low concentration of Na+ within the proximal tubule cells

Fig. 2.19 Forces governing Na$^+$ transport in the proximal tubule.

Forces governing Na$^+$ transport in the proximal tubule			
Part of proximal tubule	**Electrical potential (mV)**	**Transport mechanism**	**Na$^+$ concentration (mmol/L)**
tubular lumen	−2	passive (carrier molecule)	150
cell	−70	active (pump)	30
extracellular fluid	0	diffusion	150

Fig. 2.19 Forces governing Na$^+$ transport in the proximal tubule.

(less than 30 mmol/L) and there is also a negative transmembrane potential relative to the lumen (−70 mV). This drives Na$^+$ ions to move along their concentration and electrical gradient into the cells from the tubular fluid via carrier molecules on the apical membrane. The movement of other inorganic ions and molecules is coupled with Na$^+$ transport in and out of tubule cells:

- Glucose, amino acids, PO$_4^{3-}$ ions, and lactate are transported by symport with Na$^+$ into the cell.
- H$^+$ is transported by antiport out of the cell and linked to the reabsorption of HCO$_3^-$.

The forces governing Na$^+$ transport in the proximal tubule are shown in Fig. 2.19.

Chloride reabsorption

Over 60% of filtered Cl$^-$ is reabsorbed in the middle and late proximal tubule. Cl$^-$ enter the cells by passive reabsorption; however, the intercellular potential opposes Cl$^-$ entry into the cells in the early part of the proximal tubule. The reabsorption of glucose, amino acids, and HCO$_3^-$ with Na$^+$ in the initial part of the proximal tubule leaves behind a filtrate that becomes concentrated with Cl$^-$. The increase in Cl$^-$ produces a diffusion gradient, which allows movement of the ions into the intercellular space or directly into the cell:

- Most Cl$^-$ entry is via the tight junctions between cells along with Na$^+$.
- A small amount of Cl$^-$ enters by antiport with HCO$_3^-$ and HCOO$^-$ (formate).

Water reabsorption

80% of the filtered water is reabsorbed in the proximal tubule. This occurs as a consequence of the high Na$^+$ concentration in the lateral intercellular spaces, which is maintained by the constant removal of Na$^+$ from the cell by the Na$^+$/K$^+$ ATPase pump (Fig. 2.20). The resulting watery fluid causes an increase in the hydrostatic pressure and there is movement of fluid through the basement membrane into the peritubular capillary. This movement is favoured by the high oncotic pressure in the capillary due to the with concentration of plasma proteins created by the filtration process in the glomerulus.

The fluid leaving the proximal tubule is isosmotic as both ions and water move out of the filtrate together. The proximal tubule has no concentrating capacity.

Transport of other solutes in the proximal tubule

Glucose

The normal range for plasma glucose concentration is 2.5–5.5 mmol/L. About 0.2–0.5 mmol of glucose is filtered every minute with a normal plasma concentration. Any increase in the plasma glucose concentration results in a proportional increase in the amount of glucose filtered. Virtually all filtered glucose is reabsorbed in the proximal tubule, unless the amount of filtered glucose exceeds the resorptive capacity of the cells. Glucose is transported into the proximal tubule cells by symport (secondary active transport) against its concentration gradient. It is driven by the energy

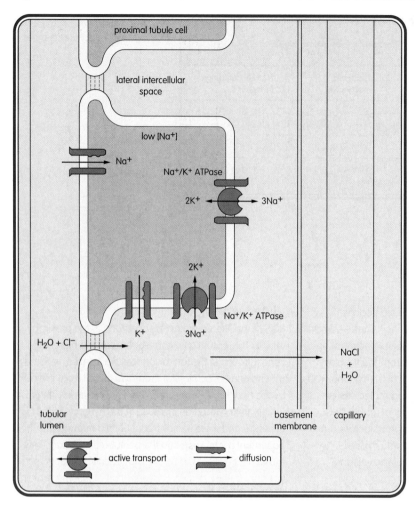

Fig. 2.20 NaCl transport in the proximal tubule.

released from the transport of Na+ down its electrochemical gradient as the Na+/K+ ATPase pump on the basolateral membrane maintains a low Na+ concentration and negative potential within the cell (Fig. 2.21). This is an example of secondary active transport. The transport ratio is:

- 1:1 Na+:glucose in the pars convoluta.
- 2:1 Na+:glucose in the pars recta.

All nephrons have different thresholds for glucose reabsorption (nephron heterogeneity). T_m is the maximum tubular resorptive capacity for a solute (i.e. the point of saturation for the carriers), and this value can be calculated for glucose. There are a limited number of Na+/glucose carrier molecules and so glucose reabsorption is T_m limited. Fig. 2.22 shows that

the lowest renal threshold of glucose is at a plasma glucose concentration of 10 mmol/L. At this level filtered glucose will begin to be excreted in the urine (glycosuria). As plasma glucose concentration increases further even the nephrons with highest resorptive capacity will allow glucose excretion and urinary glucose increases in parallel with plasma glucose. The T_m for glucose is exceeded in all nephrons when the plasma glucose concentration is greater than 20 mmol/L.

Glucose will appear in the urine (glycosuria) if either the filtered load exceeds the renal threshold or the T_m for glucose is lower than normal. In diabetes, plasma glucose is elevated and hence the filtered load of glucose increased—if glasma glucose is greater than 10 mmol/L, glycosuria will result. In certain inherited tubular disorders, T_m for glucose is low and glycosuria

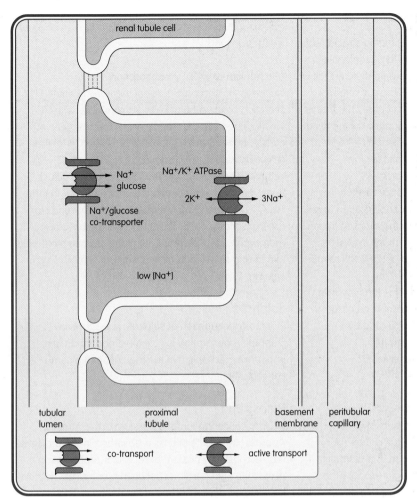

Fig. 2.21 Glucose transport in cells of the pars convoluta.

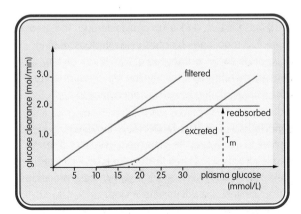

Fig. 2.22 Relationship between plasma concentration, filtration, reabsorption, and excretion of glucose. GFR is assumed to be 100 mL/min. T_m is exceeded in some nephrons with plasma glucose >10 mmol/L and for all nephrons when plasma glucose >20 mmol/L (nephron heterogeneity gives rise to 'splay' on the curve).

may be found with a normal plasma glucose (renal glycosuria)—the patient is not diabetic. Renal glycosuria may also occur in pregnancy, because T_m for glucose is reduced; however, it should be noted that true diabetes may also occur in pregnancy and cause glycosuria.

Amino acids

The plasma concentration of amino acids is 2.5–3.5 mmol/L. Amino acids are the basic unit of proteins and are constantly absorbed from the gut. They are small molecules that easily filter through the glomerulus, and most of the reabsorption occurs in the proximal tubule. The transport is by symport with Na^+ and is driven by Na^+/K^+ ATPase as with glucose. There are about five different transport classes coupled with Na^+, and these are responsible for the movement of different types of amino acid residues. This is a T_m-limited process.

Phosphate

Phosphate (PO_4^{3-}) salts are essential for the structure of bones and teeth. 80% of the body's PO_4^{3-} content is in the skeleton and 20% is in the intracellular fluid (ICF). It is easily filtered at the glomerulus: 80% is reabsorbed in the proximal tubule and the 20% of filtered PO_4^{3-} that is lost in the urine is due to the impermeability of the distal nephron to PO_4^{3-}.

The kidney is also an important site for the regulation of PO_4^{3-}. The amount filtered is proportional to the plasma PO_4^{3-} concentration. Therefore any increase in plasma concentration (over 1.2 mmol/L) leads to an increase in the amount filtered and excreted, and in this way alterations in plasma PO_4^{3-} levels can be controlled. A fall in GFR will result in increased plasma PO_4^{3-} concentration. Reabsorption of PO_4^{3-} occurs with Na^+ ions (two Na^+ with one PO_4^{3-} ion) at the apical membrane of the tubular cells. PO_4^{3-} ion uptake is regulated by parathyroid hormone (PTH) and vitamin D.

PO_4^{3-} is an important urinary buffer for H^+.

Urea

Plasma concentration of urea is normally 2.5–7.5 mmol/L. Urea is the end-product of protein metabolism, which occurs in the liver; it is then transported to the kidneys in the blood. It is a small molecule that is freely filtered at the glomerulus. The concentration of urea increases in the filtrate as a result of Na^+, Cl^-, and water removal. This then permits passive reabsorption of urea along its concentration gradient; 40–50% of the urea is absorbed in this way. 50–60% of the filtered urea is excreted in the urine. Antidiuretic hormone (ADH) increases the permeability of urea in the inner medullary collecting ducts. The distal tubule and the outer medullary ducts are impermeable to urea.

Bicarbonate

Plasma concentration of bicarbonate (HCO_3^-) is 20–30 mmol/L. HCO_3^- is vital in the maintenance of acid–base balance within the body. The kidney plays an important part in the regulation of pH by controlling the plasma HCO_3^- concentration. 90% of the filtered HCO_3^- is reabsorbed into the proximal tubule (Fig. 2.23) and the remaining 10% is taken up in the distal tubule and collecting ducts. Reabsorption of HCO_3^- is also coupled to Na^+ transport.

Mechanism of HCO_3^- reabsorption

Na^+ reabsorption on the apical membrane drives H^+ secretion by the tubular cells. H^+ combines with HCO_3^- ions to form H_2CO_3 (carbonic acid). The presence of carbonic anhydrase (CA) on the brush border of the cells catalyses the dissociation of $H_2CO_3 \rightarrow H_2O + CO_2$ within the tubular lumen. Both H_2O and CO_2 diffuse freely into the cell where they are recombined to form H_2CO_3, catalysed by intracellular CA. HCO_3^- and Na^+ are transported out of the cell across the basolateral membrane. H^+ is secreted out of the cell into the tubular lumen and recycled to allow continuation of this cycle (see Fig. 2.23).

Sulphate

Plasma concentration of sulphate is 1–1.5 mmol/L. Sulphate reabsorption is T_m limited and this is an important mechanism in the regulation of plasma concentration.

Potassium

Plasma concentration of potassium is 4–5 mmol/L. Approximately 80% of K^+ is reabsorbed in the proximal tubule, mostly by passive paracellular reabsorption across the tight junctions between tubular cells. K^+ can be secreted or reabsorbed in the nephron. The excretion can vary from 1% to 110% of the filtered K^+ depending upon the dietary intake of potassium, the acid–base status, and levels of aldosterone. The greater part of K^+ reabsorption occurs in the thick ascending loop of Henle by co-transport of $Na^+/K^+/Cl^-$ on the luminal membrane. Reabsorption of K^+ occurs in the distal tubule during severe dietary depletion of K^+.

Secretion by the proximal tubule

Secretion consists of the movement of solutes from the proximal tubule cells into the tubular fluid. It can be active (i.e. requires energy) or passive. These processes are T_m limited or gradient time limited.

There are three T_m-limited secretory mechanisms for:
- Strong organic bases (e.g. choline, histamine, guanidine, and thiamine), which are secreted in the pars convoluta.

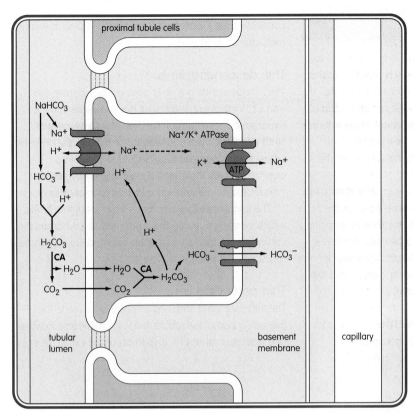

Fig. 2.23 Reabsorption of HCO_3^- ions in the proximal tubule cells. Secreted H^+ combines with HCO_3^- to form carbonic acid. This is broken down by carbonic anhydrase (CA) in the brush border to CO_2 and H_2O, which diffuse freely into the cell. The process is reveresed inside the cell to re-form HCO_3^-.

- Strong organic acids (e.g. penicillin, *p*-aminohippuric acid—PAH), which are secreted in the pars recta as the substances move out from the peritubular capillaries.
- Ethylenediaminetetraacetic acid (EDTA).

The substances handled by gradient time-limited mechanisms include:

- H^+— secretion of H^+ is related to the transport of Na^+ and the reabsorption of HCO_3^-. The movement of H^+ out of the cells occurs by an antiport with Na^+ on the apical membrane using a specific transporter.
- K^+—this is very variable and depends upon the diet, aldosterone levels, acid–base status, and the urine flow.

- Outline sodium handling by the proximal tubule.
- Describe the transport of glucose in the proximal tubule.
- Discuss the reabsorption of HCO_3^- in the proximal tubule.

LOOP OF HENLE

Role of the loop of Henle

The overall effect of the loop of Henle is reabsorption of 20% of the filtered Na^+ and 10% of tubular water. As filtrate flows through the loop of Henle, reabsorption of NaCl in the thick ascending limb produces a hypertonic interstitial fluid in the medulla. As a result of the hypertonic medulla, water moves passively out of the thin descending limb.

The tubular fluid is isotonic to the plasma on entering the loop of Henle; however, by the time it leaves the loop it is hypotonic because of reabsorption of ions within the loop. This allows urine to be concentrated with minimum energy expenditure because water is passively reabsorbed from the collecting ducts into the hypertonic interstitium of the medulla.

Structure of the loop of Henle

The different components of the loop can be considered as functionally separate units, each with its own specific properties.

Thin descending limb

The thin descending limb is permeable to water, Na^+, and Cl^-. Water reabsorption is passively driven by the hypertonic interstitium of the medulla. Movement of NaCl into the lumen and water out of the lumen into the interstitium allows the tubular fluid to come into equilibrium with the interstitium. It is lined by thin, flat cells that have minimal cytoplasmic specialization.

The juxtamedullary nephrons have long, thin limbs, which extend deep into the inner medulla, whereas the cortical nephrons only just enter the medulla and some are situated entirely in the cortex.

Thin ascending limb

The thin ascending limb has a similar structure to the preceding part of the tubule, but is impermeable to water and has minimal NaCl transport occurring within the cells.

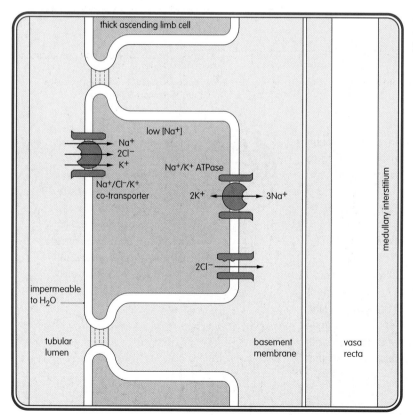

Fig. 2.24 Transport of ions in the cells of the thick ascending limb of the loop of Henle:
- $Na^+/Cl^-/K^+$ co-transporter
- Na^+/K^+ ATPase
- Cl^- channel.

Thick ascending limb

The thick ascending limb extracts Na^+ (20% of the filtered Na^+ is reabsorbed in the loop of Henle) and Cl^- ions from the tubular fluid into the interstitium. As a result the filtrate becomes progressively diluted since this part of the tubule is impermeable to water. There is co-transport (symport) of Na^+, Cl^-, and K^+ (1:2:1) (i.e. the pump is electrochemically neutral) on the apical membrane. This transport process is driven by the Na^+ gradient across the cell membrane. Na^+ is removed from the cell by the Na^+/K^+ ATPase pump on the basolateral membrane and Cl^- diffuses passively out as a result of Na^+ movement; however, most of the K^+ leaks back into the cell and tubular lumen. The net result is that NaCl accumulates in the medullary interstitium. Fig. 2.24 shows the transport of ions in the cells in the thick ascending limb of the loop of Henle.

Fig. 2.25 shows the transport processes in the loop of Henle.

Countercurrent multiplication

Any mechanism that will concentrate urine needs to have the ability to reabsorb water from the tubular fluid as it passes through the collecting ducts. This is achieved by the loop of Henle: as it acts as a countercurrent multiplier it produces a hypertonic medulla by the pooling of NaCl in the interstitium and this favours the movement of water out of the collecting ducts. The characteristics of each portion of the loop have already been discussed and they are essential to the effectiveness of this system.

A model to demonstrate the mechanism of the countercurrent multiplier is illustrated in Figs 2.26–2.29.

The thick, ascending limb can maintain a difference of 200 mOsmol/kg H_2O between the tubular fluid and the interstitium at any level, all the way along its length. The maximum osmolality of the interstitium is 1400 mOsmol/kg H_2O (normal plasma osmolality is 300 mOsmol/kg H_2O) at the tip of the loop. The fluid leaving the loop of Henle is hypotonic (100 mOsmol/kg H_2O).

Role of urea and vasa recta

The countercurrent mechanism requires an environment in which the waste products and water are cleared without disturbing the solutes that maintain the medullary hypertonicity. This countercurrent exchange is provided by the vasa recta capillary system derived from the efferent arterioles of the longer juxtaglomerular

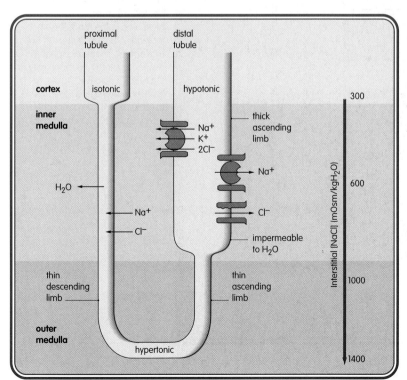

Fig. 2.25 Transport processes in the loop of Henle:
- $Na^+/Cl^-/K^+$ co-transporter
- Na^+/K^+ ATPase
- Cl^- channel.

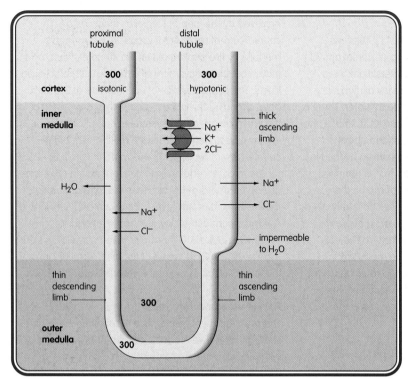

Fig. 2.26 If the whole of the loop of Henle is filled with fluid of 300 mOsmol/L (isotonic with plasma), there will be a constant concentration throughout the system (i.e. the whole system will come into equilibrium).

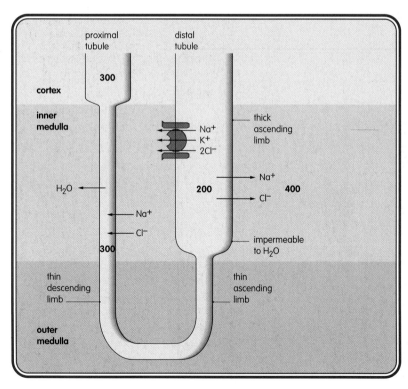

Fig. 2.27 As active resorption of Na^+, Cl^-, and K^+ occurs in the thick ascending limb, the concentration of solutes in the medulla increases. Because there is no movement of water in the thick ascending limb, the osmolality of the tubular fluid decreases (200 mOsmol/kg H_2O) and the osmolality of the interstitium increases (400 mOsmol/kg H_2O).

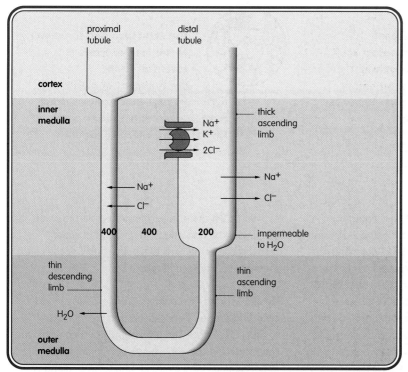

Fig. 2.28 The increase in the interstitial osmolality will cause passive movement of water out of the thin descending limb into the medullary interstitium. It also causes NaCl to move into the filtrate. This occurs until an equilibrium is reached (400 mOsmol/kg H$_2$O) between the thin, descending limb and the interstitium.

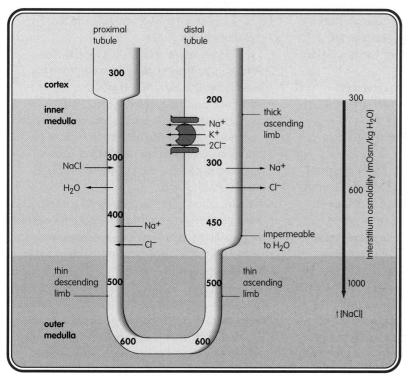

Fig. 2.29 The constant removal of NaCl will continue to decrease the osmolality of the tubular fluid in the thick ascending limb, with most resorption occurring at the tip of the loop (600 mOsmol/kg H$_2$O). This will further increase the osmolality of the fluid in the thin descending limb as it comes into equilibrium with its surroundings. In this way, a longitudinal gradient of osmolality is created in the medulla.

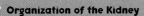

The countercurrent multiplier of the loop of Henle is an important physiological mechanism and is a common subject in exams.

The structure and function of the loop of Henle is essential to the development of medullary hypertonicity, which allows urine to be concentrated as it passes through the collecting tubules.

nephrons. It does not require metabolic energy.

The capillaries have a hairpin arrangement adjacent to the loop of Henle and are permeable to water and solutes. As the descending vessels pass through the medulla they take up solutes such as Na^+, urea, and Cl^- and water moves along its osmotic gradient out of the capillaries. At the tip of the loop the capillary blood has the same osmolality as the interstitium and an osmotic equilibrium is reached. The vessels of the vasa recta that ascend with the corresponding loop of Henle contain very viscous blood due to the loss of water from the capillaries. The increase in oncotic pressure due to concentration of plasma proteins favours the movement of water back into the blood vessel from the interstitium. However, the majority of NaCl is retained in the interstitium to maintain the hypertonic medullary environment.

The collecting tubules traverse the cortex and medulla. They consist of two functionally different parts:
• The cortical collecting ducts.
• The medullary (inner and outer) collecting ducts.

Both parts are impermeable to NaCl. The permeability to water and urea (only in the inner medullary collecting ducts) varies according to the presence of antidiuretic hormone (ADH). ADH increases the permeability to water and in this way the concentration of the urine can be controlled. The action of ADH is to increase water uptake in the cortical collecting tubules resulting in the production of a more concentrated urine.

The water reabsorbed in the medullary part of the collecting ducts is taken up by the vasa recta to prevent dilution of the medullary interstitium, which is crucial to the function of the distal nephron and the concentration of urine.

About 20% of the initial glomerular filtrate enters the distal nephron and, mainly as a result of water resbsorption in the cortical tubules, only 5% goes into the medullary collecting ducts.

Fig. 2.30 shows the countercurrent exchanger and the collecting duct as it passes through the medulla.

ADH also affects the permeability of urea within the medullary cortical tubules; however, urea remains impermeable in the cortical tubules. Urea, along with NaCl, is very important in the maintenance of medullary hypertonicity as follows:
• 50% of the filtered urea is reabsorbed in the proximal tubule with Na^+.
• The tubular concentration of urea increases as it diffuses out of the medullary interstitium into the lumen down its concentration gradient.
• The remaining urea becomes gradually more concentrated within the tubular lumen as water and other solutes are reabsorbed into the cells of the distal tubule and the cortical collecting tubules, especially since these parts of the nephron are impermeable to urea.
• In the medullary collecting tubules the concentration of urea is so high that it diffuses out of the lumen into the interstitium, thus increasing the concentration of urea in the medulla and recycling it. This occurs in the presence of ADH.

A high-protein diet increases the amount of urea in the blood for excretion as a result of increased metabolism and consequently there is more urea in the medullary interstitium and a higher urinary osmolality can be achieved.

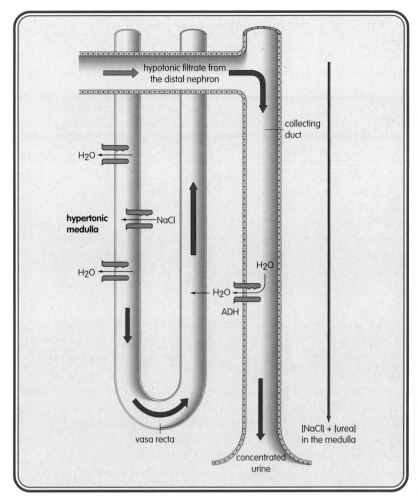

Fig. 2.30 Countercurrent exchanger as it passes through the medulla. The descending vessels of the vasa recta lose water as they pass through the hypertonic medulla. As a result of increasing oncotic pressure in the ascending vessels, water is passively reabsorbed back into the blood vessels from the interstitium as water uptake occurs in the collecting ducts under the influence of ADH. Because of this uptake of water by the vasa recta, the high osmolality of the medullary interstitium is maintained and this hypertonic environment allows continued concentration of the tubular fluid in the collecting duct.

Regulation of urine concentration

The levels of ADH within the body determine the concentration and volume of urine:

- Average daily urine volume is 1.0–1.5 L (range 400 mL to 23 L).
- Average urine osmolality is 450 mOsmol/kg H_2O (range 60–1400 mOsmol/kg H_2O).

The presence of cortisol is vital for the action of ADH. Aldosterone is also very important in concentrating urine and it does this by affecting Na^+ resorption. By increasing uptake of Na^+ in the cortical collecting tubules water reabsorption increases and urine volume decreases and osmolality increases (see Chapter 3 for a detailed discussion of ADH).

Urine can be diluted and concentrated over a wide range to allow for changes in water intake and non-renal losses.

- Outline the countercurrent mechanism of the loop of Henle.
- How does ADH affect urine concentration?

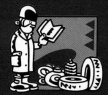

3. Renal Function

RENAL BLOOD FLOW AND THE GLOMERULAR FILTRATION RATE (GFR)

Plasma creatinine is commonly used as an indicator of renal function.

Measurement of the GFR

Clearance

Clearance (C) is the volume of plasma, that is cleared of a substance in unit time or an assessment of the ability of the kidney to remove a substance from the plasma and excrete it. If x = substance cleared, P_x = concentration of that substance in arterial plasma (mg/mL), U_x = concentration of the substance in the urine (mg/mL), and V = production rate of urine (mL/min):

$$C_x = \frac{U_x \times V}{P_x}$$

Clearance of a substance that 'follows' the filtrate and is not reabsorbed, secreted, synthesized, or metabolized by the kidney provides a good estimate of the GFR. Clearance of such a substance is used to assess renal function in disease. Inulin is such a substance:

- It is a polysaccharide of molecular weight 5500.
- It is not a normal constituent of the body and is introduced into the body by injection or intravenous infusion.
- It passes through the glomerular filtrate, but is not reabsorbed, secreted, synthesized, or metabolized by the kidney; therefore all inulin filtered by the glomerulus is excreted in the urine.

Normal inulin clearance is 125 mL/min/1.73 m² body surface area (varies with body size). This is the GFR.

Creatinine clearance is used as an estimate of GFR. Creatinine is a normal constituent of the body, being a product of muscle metabolism:

$$\text{Phosphocreatine} + \text{ADP} \xrightarrow{\text{creatine phosphokinase}} \text{Creatine} + \text{ATP}$$
$$\text{Creatine} + H_2O \longrightarrow \text{Creatinine}$$

If renal function, muscle mass and metabolism are stable, plasma creatinine levels are constant. Plasma creatinine is a commonly used indicator of renal

function. It has a reciprocal relationship with GFR, the exact nature depending upon muscle mass and therefore age, sex, and size. The relationship between plasma creatinine and GFR is shown in Fig. 3.1.

Like inulin, creatinine is freely filtered and not reabsorbed, synthesized, or metabolized by the kidney. Therefore it can be used to measure GFR. However, some creatinine is secreted by the tubules, which can slightly affect GFR measurement. This is thought to be cancelled out by inaccuracies in the measurement of creatinine, which overestimate the true plasma creatinine concentration. Exercise affects creatinine levels and can therefore affect GFR measurements.

Clearance ratios

Information about how the kidney clears a solute can be obtained by comparison with the clearance of inulin:

- Substances with clearance values greater than those

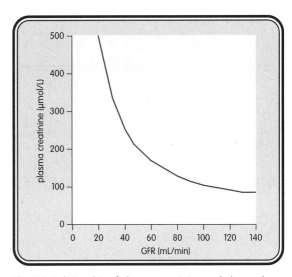

Fig. 3.1 Relationship of plasma creatinine and glomerular filtration rate (GFR). (From Renal Physiology, 2nd Edition. BM Koeppen, B Stanton. Mosby Year Book, 1996.)

for inulin clearance—the solute gets into the renal tubule by glomerular filtration and tubular secretion (e.g. PAH—*p*-aminohippuric acid).

- Substances with clearance values lower than those for inulin clearance—these are either substances that are not freely filtered at the glomerulus or substances that are freely filtered and then reabsorbed from the tubule.

Measurement of renal blood flow

The Fick principle states that where RPF = renal plasma flow; A_x = arterial concentration of a substance; V_x = venous concentration; U_x = urinary concentration; and V = urinary flow rate:

$$(RPF \times A_x) - (RPF \times V_x) = V \times U_x$$

For a substance with an extraction of 100%, $V_x = 0$ and the above simplifies to:

$$RPF \times A_x = V \times U_x$$

or,

$$RPF = \frac{V \times U_x}{P_x} = C_x$$

PAH is an organic acid. Excretion results from secretion [transport maximum (T_m) limited] by the proximal tubule and filtration at the glomerulus. If the T_m for PAH is not exceeded, the extraction approaches 100% (90% or more) in a normal individual. Therefore the clearance of PAH can be used to measure RPF (Fig. 3.2). When plasma PAH concentration is less than 0.1 mg/mL, T_m for PAH is not exceeded, the extraction of PAH approaches 100% and C_{PAH} equals renal plasma flow.

When the excretion of PAH is 100%, if P_{PAH} is the plasma concentration of PAH, U_{PAH} is the urine concentration of PAH, and V is urinary flow rate:

$$RPF \times P_{PAH} = V \times U_{PAH}$$

or,

$$RPF = \frac{V \times U_{PAH}}{P_{PAH}} = C_{PAH}$$

RPF is typically 600 mL/min.

Renal blood flow (RBF) can be obtained from RPF by using the haematocrit. The haematocrit is 45%, therefore plasma is 55%:

$$
\begin{aligned}
RBF &= RPF \times 100/55 \\
&= 600 \times 100/55 \\
&= 1100 \, mL/min
\end{aligned}
$$

However, C_{PAH} is not an exact measurement of RPF. This is because blood goes not only to the glomeruli and tubules, but also to the capsule, perirenal fat, and medulla. Therefore, PAH approximates cortical plasma flow and is usually referred to as effective RPF (ERPF).

If extraction of PAH is reduced significantly C_{PAH} becomes a less reliable marker of RPF unless allowance is made for decreased extraction. This occurs:

- When [PAH] is greater than T_m.
- In chronic renal failure.
- In tubular dysfunction.

Other methods of measuring RBF

Inert gas 'washout' technique

Radioactive krypton (^{84}Kr) or xenon (^{133}Xe) is injected into the renal artery with a small amount of saline. The gas diffuses throughout the kidneys almost immediately at a rate dependent upon RBF. Therefore, the rate of removal of gas from the kidneys can be used to determine RBF.

Isotope uptake technique

Radioactive potassium (^{42}K) or rubidium (^{86}Rb) is given intravenously. The amount of isotope in different parts of the kidney gives an indication of the blood flow through the kidney. This method requires removal of the kidneys and is only applicable to experimental studies in animals.

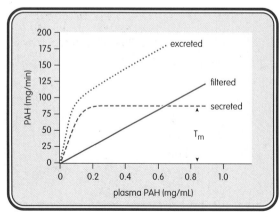

Fig. 3.2 Filtration, excretion, and secretion of *p*-aminohippuric acid (PAH) compared with its plasma concentration.

Filtration fraction

This is the percentage of plasma flow filtered through the glomeruli into the nephrons:

Filtration fraction = GFR/RPF

In a normal man:

Filtration fraction = 125/600

= 20%

Fractional excretion (FE)

This is a measure of net reabsorption or net secretion of a substance:

FE_x = mass excreted/mass filtered

= $(U_x \times V)/(GFR \times P_x)$

FE is often expressed as a percentage. Therefore, if the FE is 0.24, 24% of the filtered mass is excreted and 76% undergoes net reabsorption.

Regulation of RBF and GFR

- RBF is 1100 mL/min
- GFR is 125 mL/min.

Both vary very little because of autoregulation (Fig. 3.3). Over a wide range of perfusion pressures (e.g. 90–200 mmHg), blood flow is independent of perfusion pressure; therefore, as perfusion pressure increases, resistance to flow increases. Tone in both afferent and efferent arterioles can be altered, to maintain constant RBF and GFR (Fig. 3.4). How these techniques work is not clear. The following mechanisms have been proposed:

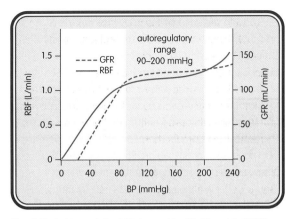

Fig. 3.3 Autoregulation of glomerular filtration rate (GFR) and renal blood flow (RBF).

- Myogenic theory.
- Tubuloglomerular feedback mechanism.

Myogenic theory

An increase in pressure stimulates stretch receptors in vascular smooth muscle, thereby increasing Ca^{2+} and increasing tension of the afferent arteriole. This results in contraction of smooth muscle fibres in the vessel wall and increased resistance to flow, thus keeping flow constant.

Tubuloglomerular feedback mechanism

This has three main mediating mechanisms:

- Angiotensin II (locally formed).
- Prostaglandins.
- Adenosine (potent vasoconstrictor).

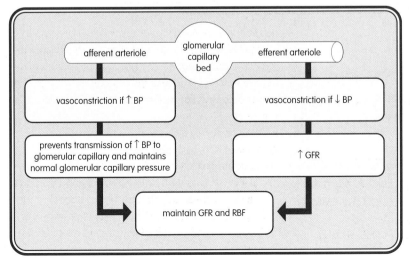

Fig. 3.4 Regulation of renal blood flow (RBF) and glomerular filtration rate (GFR) by vasoconstriction of arterioles.

The macula densa (a dense body that detects pressure/flow changes within the kidney) detects changes in Na+ flow, possibly by a mechanism dependent on reabsorption. Changes in the pressure/flow are transmitted from the macula densa to granular cells. (There is a close association between granular cells containing renin and the macula densa.) This leads to the production of angiotensin II, which then causes vasoconstriction. Prostaglandins and adenosine play a small part in this mechanism.

Renal blood flow and systemic blood pressure

Autoregulation maintains the blood flow to the kidneys despite changes in the blood pressure. The blood flow is, however, not always constant—for example haemorrhage results in increased sympathetic activity to the kidney (and other parts of the body), which in turn leads to vasoconstriction and decreased blood flow by response to such events. Intrarenal vasodilator prostaglandins are produced to prevent excessive vasoconstriction and renal perfusion is thus maintained.

Regulation of GFR involves other vasoactive substances, which are found in the walls of blood vessels such as:
- Endothelin—a potent vasoconstrictor.
- Nitric oxide (NO)—a potent vasodilator.

Age-related changes in RBF and GFR

Age-related changes in RBF and GFR (Fig. 3.5) are as follows:
- 10th week of gestation—filtration of fluid and urine production commence.
- Postpartum—GFR ≈ 25 mL/min/1.73 m² body surface area.
- Newborn—RBF ≈ 5% of cardiac output; increases progressively during the first year.
- 1 month old—progressive increase in GFR. (PAH cannot be used to measure RBF as tubular secretion is not developed and therefore extraction of PAH is less than 100%.)
- By 1 year of age—GFR reaches adult value (125 mL/min).
- Adults—RBF ≈ 20% of cardiac output.
- Old age—GFR decreases.

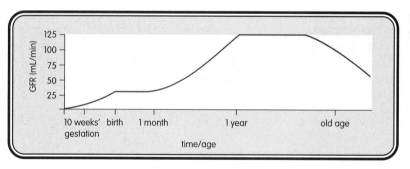

Fig. 3.5 Age-related changes in glomerular filtration rate (GFR).

- What is clearance? How is it measured and what are its units? What are clearance ratios?
- How do you measure the GFR and RBF? How does this vary with age?
- What factors affect creatinine clearance?
- What is autoregulation and how is it achieved?

BODY FLUID OSMOLALITY

Concepts of osmolality

Body weight remains relatively constant from day to day as fluid volume remains constant. In Chapter 1, the normal intake and output of water are discussed. A urine output of at least 400 mL/day is required for the kidney to maintain homeostasis.

The normal plasma osmolality (P_{osm}) is 280–290 mosmol/kg H_2O. This is very strictly regulated and an increase or decrease of 3 mosmol/kg H_2O) will stimulate the body's osmolality regulation mechanism.

Osmoreceptors

Osmoreceptors detect changes in the plasma osmolality, and are located in the supraoptic and

An excess of water reduces plasma osmolality.
Water deficiency increases plasma osmolality.

paraventricular areas of the anterior hypothalamus. Their blood supply is the internal carotid artery. They regulate the release of antidiuretic hormone (ADH, also known as vasopressin). Thirst is regulated by these osmoreceptors and others in the lateral preoptic area of the hypothalamus. Fig. 3.6 illustrates the role of ADH in maintaining osmolality.

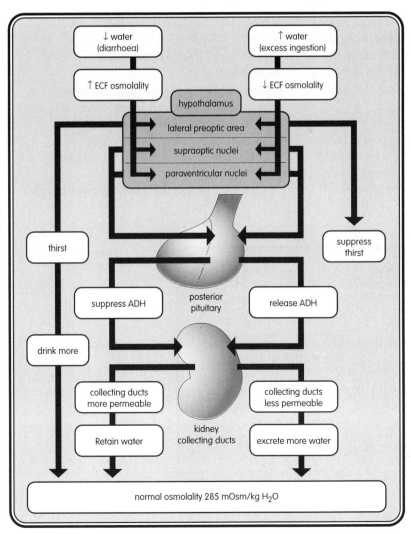

Fig. 3.6 Role of antidiuretic hormone (ADH) in maintaining osmolality. (ECF, extracellular fluid.)

Sensitivity of osmoreceptors to osmotic changes caused by different solutes

Na^+ and other associated anions are the main constituents that determine plasma osmolality. Water loss alters the Na^+ concentration. Other solutes without the addition or loss of water can also change the osmolality. Not all solutes equally stimulate the osmoreceptors. The amount they do varies depending upon how easily they can cross the cell membranes (i.e. their ability to cause cellular dehydration).

ADH (antidiuretic hormone)

Synthesis and storage

ADH is synthesized in the supraoptic nucleus of the hypothalamus as large precursor molecules and is transported to the neurohypophysis (Fig. 3.7).

Release

ADH release occurs in response to increased plasma osmolality. This leads to action potentials in the neurons from the hypothalamus (contains ADH), which depolarize the cell membrane, resulting in Ca^{2+} influx, fusion of secretory granules with the cell membrane, and release of ADH and neurophysin.

Cellular actions

When present on the peritubular side of the collecting tubule cell (Fig. 3.8), ADH causes an increase in water permeability by the insertion of water channels (aquaporins) into the luminal membrane. It is not effective if present on the luminal side. This is because ADH receptors (V_2 receptors) are on the basal membrane of the tubular cells. The V_2 receptors are G-protein coupled receptors, which have a seven membrane-spanning region. Urine osmolality (mosmol/kg) in relation to plasma ADH concentration is shown in Fig. 3.9.

Fate of ADH

ADH must be rapidly removed from the blood. This occurs in the liver and kidneys (50%), with less than 10% appearing in the urine. The rest is metabolized. Plasma half-life of ADH is 10–15 min.

Drugs affecting ADH release

Drugs may:
- Increase ADH release (e.g. nicotine, ether, morphine, barbiturates).
- Inhibit ADH release (e.g. alcohol).

Syndrome of inappropriate ADH (SIADH) secretion

Occasionally ADH is secreted inappropriately by the pituitary or other areas in the body. Causes are given in Fig. 3.10. Signs and symptoms are:
- Hyponatraemia and hypo-osmolality.
- Inappropriate urine osmolality (i.e. not maximally diluted).
- Continued natriuresis—urinary Na over 20 mmol/L

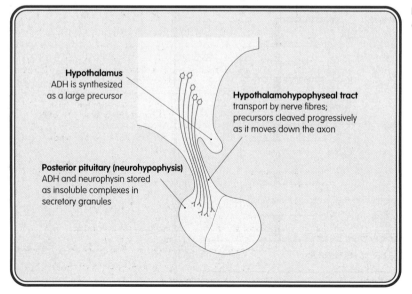

Fig. 3.7 Synthesis and storage of antidiuretic hormone (ADH).

Hypothalamus
ADH is synthesized as a large precursor

Hypothalamohypophyseal tract
transport by nerve fibres; precursors cleaved progressively as it moves down the axon

Posterior pituitary (neurohypophysis)
ADH and neurophysin stored as insoluble complexes in secretory granules

despite a decrease in plasma Na^+ concentration because the plasma volume is maintained by water retention (unless volume contracted or sodium restricted, which can decrease urinary Na^+).

The diagnosis should be considered in hyponatraemic patients in the absence of hypovolemia, oedema, endocrine dysfunction, renal failure, and drugs, all of which may impair water excretion.

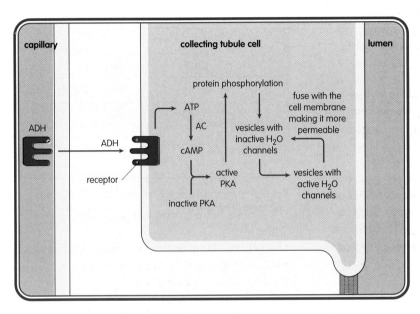

Fig. 3.8 Actions of antidiuretic hormone (ADH) in the collecting tubule. (AC, adenylate cyclase; cAMP, cyclic adenosine monophosphate; PKA, protein kinase.)

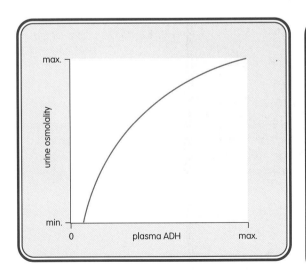

Fig. 3.9 Urine osmolality in relation to plasma antidiuretic hormone (ADH) concentration. (From Physiology, 3rd edition. RM Berne, MN Levy. Mosby Year Book, 1996.)

Causes of SIADH	
Disorder	**Example of finding**
CNS disorders	abscess, stroke, vasculitis (systemic lupus erythematosus)
malignancy	small cell carcinoma in lungs, duodenum, pancreas, prostate, ureter, adrenals
lung diseases	tuberculosis, pneumonia, abscess, aspergillosis
drugs	opiates, chlorpropamide, psychotropics, cytotoxics, narcotics, oxytocin
metabolic diseases	porphyria, hypothyroidism
miscellaneous	pain (postoperative), Guillain–Barré syndrome, trauma

Fig. 3.10 Causes of SIADH (syndrome of inappropriate antidiuretic hormone secretion).

Diabetes insipidus

This is the inability to reabsorb water from the distal part of the nephron, due to the failure of secretion or action of ADH. Symptoms are:

- Polyuria.
- Polydipsia.
- Low urine osmolality.

The causes of diabetes insipidus are:

- Neurogenic/central—absence of production of ADH by the hypothalamus, which may be congenital or caused by hypothalamic damage or tumours or pituitary tumours. Can be cured by administering ADH.
- Nephrogenic—failure of the kidneys to respond to ADH, which may be due to mutations in the gene coding for V_2 receptors, pyelonephritis, polycystic kidneys, or drugs such as lithium.

Diabetes insipidus can be difficult to differentiate from psychogenic polydypsia in which large volumes of dilute urine are produced secondary to compulsive water drinking. This causes a decrease in the urine concentrating ability due to loss of medullary tonicity.

Fig. 3.11 summarizes the action of ADH.

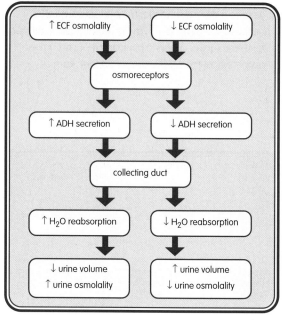

Fig. 3.11 Summary of antidiuretic hormone (ADH) action. (ECF, extracellular fluid.)

Fig. 3.12 Osmotic clearance.

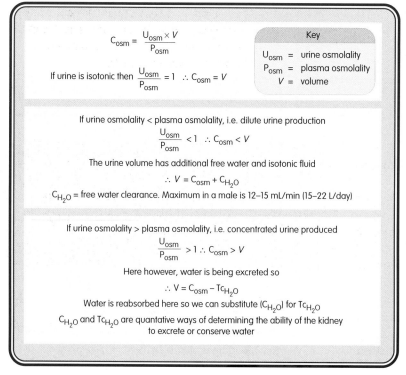

$$C_{osm} = \frac{U_{osm} \times V}{P_{osm}}$$

If urine is isotonic then $\frac{U_{osm}}{P_{osm}} = 1 \;\; \therefore C_{osm} = V$

Key

U_{osm}	=	urine osmolality
P_{osm}	=	plasma osmolality
V	=	volume

If urine osmolality < plasma osmolality, i.e. dilute urine production

$$\frac{U_{osm}}{P_{osm}} < 1 \;\; \therefore C_{osm} < V$$

The urine volume has additional free water and isotonic fluid

$$\therefore V = C_{osm} + C_{H_2O}$$

C_{H_2O} = free water clearance. Maximum in a male is 12–15 mL/min (15–22 L/day)

If urine osmolality > plasma osmolality, i.e. concentrated urine produced

$$\frac{U_{osm}}{P_{osm}} > 1 \therefore C_{osm} > V$$

Here however, water is being excreted so

$$\therefore V = C_{osm} - Tc_{H_2O}$$

Water is reabsorbed here so we can substitute (C_{H_2O}) for Tc_{H_2O}

C_{H_2O} and Tc_{H_2O} are quantative ways of determining the ability of the kidney to excrete or conserve water

Water clearance and reabsorption

Dehydration results in increased plasma osmolality. In turn the kidneys reabsorb osmotically 'free' (i.e. no solutes) water from the tubules. This results in the production of a more dilute plasma and a concentrated urine.

Ingestion of excess water results in decreased plasma osmolality. In turn the kidneys excrete osmotically 'free' water from the tubules, producing dilute urine. (Dilute urine has a lower osmolality than plasma, concentrated urine has a higher osmolality than plasma, isotonic urine has the same osmolality as plasma.) The rate at which osmotically active substances are cleared from the plasma is the osmotic clearance (C_{osm}—see p. 39). If urine is isotonic, C_{osm} = urine flow (Fig. 3.12).

Effect of solute output on urine volume

The concentrating ability of the kidneys is limited (maximum urinary osmolality is 1400 mosmol/kg). Thus the amount or urine excreted per day depends upon:

- Amount of ADH (Fig. 3.13).
- Amount of solute excreted.

At maximum ADH concentration, large amounts of solutes can still cause a diuresis (see Fig. 3.13).

Mannitol is a non-reabsorbable osmotic diuretic. It impairs renal concentrating ability and produces isotonic urine. In diabetes mellitus, the excess blood glucose causes an osmotic diuresis.

Adrenal steroids and urinary dilution

Adrenal insufficiency leads to impaired water excretion. This may reflect both mineralocorticoid and gluucocorticoid deficiency:

- Glucocorticoid deficiency may enhance water permeability of the collecting duct.
- Glucocorticoid and mineralocorticoid deficiencies increase ADH levels—the net effect is the inability to produce dilute urine. The defect is corrected by administering adrenal steroids.

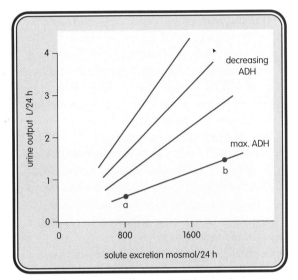

Fig. 3.13 Effect of antidiuretic hormone (ADH) on urine output. a, minimum possible urine output with a solute excretion of 800 mosmol/24 h; b, minimum urine output if 2000 mosmol/24 h must be excreted. (From Principles of Renal Physiology by C Lote, 1993.)

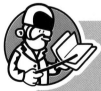

- ○ **What are osmoreceptors, where are they located, and what is their function?**
- ○ **Where is ADH synthesized and stored, how is it released, and what is its action?**
- ○ **How can the kidneys' ability to concentrate or dilute urine be altered in disease?**

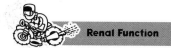

BODY FLUID VOLUME

Basic concepts
Effective circulating volume
The volume of fluid that perfuses tissues is the effective circulating volume, which needs to be maintained. Na^+ is the major extracellular ion and affects the ECF volume—for example increased ECF Na^+ results in increased osmolality, which in turn results in water retention and thirst (increased drinking of water). This increases ECF volume and normalizes osmolality. Therefore by controlling the body's Na^+, the ECF volume will be regulated.

If ECF volume decreases sufficiently, intrarenal mechanisms may decrease GFR to prevent further volume loss (tubuloglomerular feedback).

Renin and angiotensin
Renin–angiotensin–aldosterone system
The renin–angiotensin–aldosterone system (Fig. 3.14) maintains Na^+ balance.

Na^+ controls the ECF volume.

Renin
Renin is an enzyme that is synthesized and stored in the juxtaglomerular apparatus (JGA) in the kidneys. A decrease in sodium leads to a decreased ECF volume causing the release of renin by:

- Increased sympathetic innervation—decreased ECF volume results in decreased blood pressure (detected by baroreceptors in carotid arteries) and causes increased sympathetic activity. Granular cells of the JGA are innervated by the sympathetic system, so an increase in sympathetic activity leads to an increase in renin release. The process is mediated by β-adrenergic receptors.
- Decrease in the wall tension in afferent arterioles—decreased ECF volume results in decreased blood pressure which in turn decreases perfusion pressure to the kidneys. Changes in the blood pressure decrease wall tension at granular cells, resulting in increased renin release.
- Decreased Na^+ to the macula densa—decreased NaCl delivery to the macula densa stimulates the macula densa, resulting in PGI_2 secretion. PGI_2 acts on the granular cells to cause renin release.

Conversion of angiotensinogen to angiotensin
The renin that is released acts on angiotensinogen (α_2-globulin), which splits off angiotensin I (a decapeptide). Angiotensin converting enzyme (ACE) in the lungs then removes two amino acids to produce angiotensin II (an octapeptide). ACE inhibitors can be used in the treatment of high blood pressure. They decrease the production of angiotensin II and hence:
- Decrease vasoconstriction.
- Decrease aldosterone (and prevent an increase in ECF volume).

Angiotensin II:
- Acts on the zona glomerulosa of the adrenal cortex causing release of aldosterone.

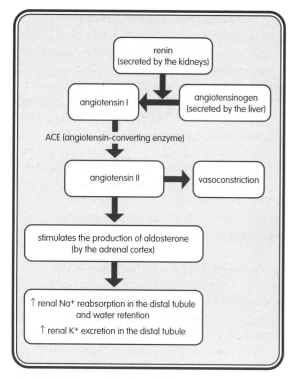

Fig. 3.14 Renin–angiotensin–aldosterone system.

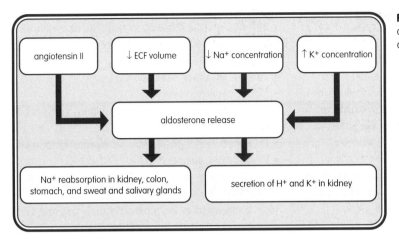

Fig. 3.15 Factors causing aldosterone release and the effects of aldosterone.

- Directly vasoconstricts arterioles within the kidney (efferent > afferent).
- Directly increases Na⁺ reabsorption from the proximal tubule.
- Releases ADH.
- Stimulates thirst.
- Provides negative feedback on the JGA cells and therefore renin release.

In addition to the generation of circulating angiotensin II, the local generation of angiotensin II by tissue ACE may be of great pathogenic importance.

Aldosterone

Aldosterone is synthesized by zona glomerulosa cells in the adrenal cortex. It is important for Na⁺ regulation and its release (Fig. 3.15) is controlled by:

- Angiotensin II.
- ECF volume—a decrease in Na⁺ decreases effective circulating volume, which then causes aldosterone release via the renin–angiotensin–aldosterone system.
- Na⁺ concentration—via the above route and also direct aldosterone release from the adrenal cortex.
- K⁺ concentration—stimulates direct release of aldosterone release from the adrenal cortex, which in turn returns K⁺ to normal by increasing distal tubular secretion of K⁺.

Cellular effects of aldosterone are:
- Promotion of Na⁺ reabsorption in the kidney, colon, gastric glands, ducts of sweat and salivary glands.
- Promotion of K⁺ and H⁺ secretion by the kidney.

Factors affecting Na⁺ reabsorption
Starling forces in the proximal tubule
The amount of Na⁺ and water uptake into the peritubular capillaries from the proximal tubule depends upon the rate and amount of uptake from the lateral intercellular spaces into the capillaries.

Changes in the body fluid volume change plasma hydrostatic and oncotic pressure—for example increased NaCl intake increases ECF volume. This in turn leads to increased hydrostatic pressure and decreased oncotic pressure and therefore decreased NaCl and water reabsorption by the proximal tubule cells.

An increase in ECF volume affects the venous pressure rather than the arterial pressure.

Sympathetic drive from the renal nerves
The arterial baroreceptors regulate renal sympathetic nerve activity; for example, decreased ECF volume decreases blood pressure, which is sensed by baroreceptors, and results in an increase in sypathetic activity. This leads to Na⁺ retention and an increase in peripheral resistance and hence restore ECF volume and blood pressure.

Increased sympathetic nerve activity to the kidney results in renin release either directly or as a result of renal vasoconstriction causing activation of JGA. Catcholamines from sympathetic nerve endings also stimulate Na^+ reabsorption by the proximal tubule, but whether this is a direct affect or secondary to altered peritubular forces is unclear.

Prostaglandins

A decrease in the effective circulating volume causes an increase in cortical prostaglandin (PG) synthesis. In the kidney PGs are synthesized in:
- The cortex (arterioles and glomeruli).
- Medullary interstitial cells.
- Collecting duct epithelial cells.

There is a variety of prostaglandins—PGE_2 (medullary), PGI_2 (cortical), $PGF_2\alpha$, PGD_2, and TXA_2 (thromboxane). Certain functions are given below:
- PGE_2, PGI_2—vasodilators, preventing excessive vasoconstriction.
- PGI_2—renin release.
- PGE_2 (medullary)—natriuretic and diuretic (collecting tubules), impairing the action of ADH, thus limiting the amount of Na^+ reabsorption in the renal medulla. PGE_2 protects the medullary tubule cells from excessive hypoxia during a decrease in ECF volume.
- TXA_2—a vasoconstrictor, which is synthesized after many renal insults (e.g. ureteral obstruction) and decreases the amount of blood available for filtration by a poorly functioning kidney.

Atrial natriuretic peptide (ANP)

ANP is a precursor produced by cardiac atrial cells. It is found in the plasma and atrial cells. An increase in ECF volume causes ANP release. ANP binds to specific cell surface receptors, resulting in increased cyclic guanosine monosulphate (cGMP). ANP:

- Inhibits Na^+/K^+ ATPase and closes Na^+ channels of the collecting ducts resulting in decreased Na^+ reabsorption.
- Inhibits aldosterone secretion.
- Decreases renin release.
- Vasodilates afferent arterioles, resulting in increased GFR.
- Decreases Na^+ reabsorption in the proximal tubules.
- Inhibits ADH release.

Dopamine

This is synthesized by the proximal tubule cells and:
- Inhibits Na^+/K^+ ATPase and Na^+/H^+ antiport, therefore decreasing tubular Na^+ transport.
- Vasodilates.
- Increases Na^+ excretion (natriuresis).

Kinins

Kallikrein cleaves kininogens to form kinins. The effects of kinins are:
- Vasodilation.
- Inhibition of ADH release.
- Increased Na^+ excretion.

Natriurietic hormone

This hormone is probably produced by the hypothalamus. It is an Na^+/K^+ ATPase inhibitor.

Fig. 3.16 illustrates the mechanisms involved in the regulation of body fluid.

REGULATION OF BODY FLUID pH

The pH in body fluid compartments is tightly controlled because most enzyme reactions are sensitive to pH changes. The normal pH range is 7.35–7.45 and H^+ concentration, 35–45 nmol/L.

- ° **Summarize the effects of the renin–angiotensin–aldosterone system.**
- ° **Outline the mechanisms controlling Na^+ reabsorption.**
- ° **How is ECF volume regulated?**

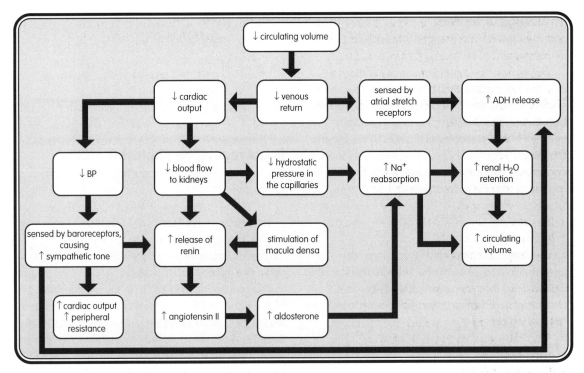

Fig. 3.16 Regulation of body fluid.

Buffers

Definition

A buffer is a mixture of a weak acid and a conjugate base that undergoes minimal pH changes when either an acid or a base is added to it:

$$HA \leftrightarrow H^+ \text{ (acid)} + A^- \text{ (conjugate base)}$$

It can also be a mixture of a weak base and conjugate acid:

$$BH^+ \leftrightarrow H^+ \text{ (conjugate acid)} + B^- \text{ (base)}$$

For example, if there is an increase in H^+, the equations above shift to the left so that the increase in H^+ combines with the buffer and the H^+ concentration in the body decreases.

The bicarbonate buffer system is an important buffering system in the body.

pK values and equilibrium constants

The equations below demonstrate the equilibrium constants in terms of conjugate acids and bases, proton donors, and acceptors.

$$HA \leftrightarrow H^+ + A^-$$

Equation 1. At equilibrium.

$$K = \frac{[H^+][A^-]}{[HA]}$$

$$\therefore [H^+] = \frac{K[HA]}{[A^-]}$$

$$= \frac{K[acid]}{[base]}$$

Equation 2.

$$pH = -\log[H^+]$$

$$= \log \frac{1}{[H^+]}$$

$$pK = -\log K$$

$$= \log \frac{1}{K}$$

Equation 3. Combining equations 1 and 2.

$$pH = pK + \log \frac{[base]}{[acid]}$$

(Henderson–Hasselbalch equation)

51

Physiological buffers

There are several buffer systems in the different body compartments (Fig. 3.17).

Bicarbonate buffer system

The bicarbonate buffer system is important in all body fluids. Carbon dioxide (CO_2) and water (H_2O) are combined to form carbonic acid (H_2CO_3) by the enzyme carbonic anhydrase (CA). The H_2CO_3 then spontaneously dissociates to form bicarbonate ions (HCO_3^-) and H^+. This is summarized in the equation below:

$$CO_2 + H_2O \xleftarrow{\text{carbonic anhydrase}} H_2CO_3 \leftrightarrow H^+ + HCO_3^-$$

CO_2 concentration is regulated by the lungs and HCO_3^- concentration is regulated by the kidneys. Therefore pH regulation depends equally on both these organs. Substituting this equation in the Henderson–Hasselbalch equation, we get:

$$pH = pK + \log [HCO_3^-]/[H_2CO_3]$$

$[H_2CO_3]$ is determined by dissolved CO_2:

$$[H_2CO_3] = 0.23 \times pCO_2 \text{ [0.23 is the } CO_2 \text{ solubility coefficient at 37°C.]}$$

Therefore, $pH = pK + \log[HCO_3^-]/0.03 \times pCO_2$

Normal values are:
- $[HCO_3^-]$—24–25 mmol/L.

- pCO_2—5.3 kPa.
- pK of HCO_3^-/pCO_2 system is 6.1.

Therefore pH = 7.4.
  In summary:

$$pH \propto HCO_3^- / pCO_2$$

Renal regulation of plasma HCO_3^-

Metabolism results in H^+ production, which in turn results in:

$$H^+ + HCO_3^- \leftrightarrow H_2CO_3 \leftrightarrow H_2O + CO_2$$

CO_2 is exhaled by the lungs. The kidneys retain HCO_3^- and make more HCO_3^-.

The concentration of HCO_3^- in the plasma filtered by the kidney is 25 mmol/L. HCO_3^- is reabsorbed by the kidney using a T_m-dependent mechanism (Fig. 3.18). The T_m is similar to the amount of HCO_3^- filtered at a normal plasma concentration. Therefore if HCO_3^- increases, T_m is exceeded, resulting in HCO_3^- excretion until the plasma level returns to normal. Fig. 3.18 illustrates the way in which HCO_3^- is handled by the kidney.

In the proximal tubule, 90% of HCO_3^- is absorbed (see Fig. 2.23 in Chapter 2).

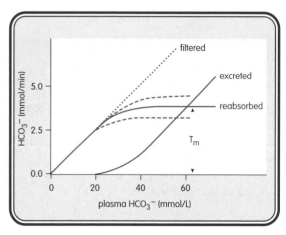

Fig. 3.18 How HCO_3^- ions are handled by the kidney. HCO_3^- absorption is dependent on H^+ secretion into the tubule. This dependancy causes the T_m for HCO_3^- absorption to vary. The limits of the T_m variability are illustrated by the dotted lines on the graph above. (From Principles of Renal Physiology by C Lote, 1993.)

Buffer systems in different body compartments			
Buffer systems	**Blood**	**ECF and CSF**	**ICF**
HCO_3^-/CO_2	X	X	X
haemoglobin	X		
plasma proteins	X		
phosphate	X	X	X
organic phosphate			X
proteins		X	X

Fig. 3.17 Buffer systems in different body compartments. (CSF, cerebrospinal fluid; ECF, extracellular fluid; ICF, intracellular fluid.)

HCO₃⁻ reabsorption

In the lumen of the proximal tubule

HCO_3^- reacts with H^+ (delivered into the lumen via an antiport process coupled with Na^+) to give H_2CO_3. H_2CO_3 dissociates into H_2O and CO_2, catalysed by an enzyme CA (present in the brush border of luminal cells). CA inhibitors inhibit the secretion of H^+, causing a decrease in the absorption of Na^+ and HCO_3^- and have a weak diuretic action.

In the tubular cells of the proximal tubule

H_2O and CO_2 enter the tubular cells and again catalysed by CA form H_2CO_3. H_2CO_3 again dissociates into:

- H^+, which is secreted into the lumen.
- HCO_3^-, which enters the plasma via the peritubular fluid (see also Fig. 2.23).

Some HCO_3^- couples with luminal Cl^- so that HCO_3^- is secreted into the lumen and Cl^- is absorbed.

In the distal nephron

Intercalated cells are involved. Secreted H^+ and luminal HCO_3^- are present, but there is not much CA. Therefore little CO_2 and H_2O are produced, resulting in less HCO_3^- absorption. H^+ ions are secreted across into the lumen by H^+ ATPase and H^+/K^+ ATPase (pumps H^+ out, K^+ in).

Conversion of alkaline phosphate to acid phosphate—luminal buffer

Both alkaline phosphate Na_2HPO_4 and acid phosphate NaH_2PO_4 are present in the plasma in the ratio of 4:1. Both are filtered at the glomerulus. Alkaline phosphate is converted to acid phosphate—mainly in the distal tubule, but some in the proximal tubule (Fig. 3.19). The important result is that HCO_3^- is generated for the plasma.

Ammonia secretion—luminal buffer

In the proximal tubule, deamination of glutamine produces ammonium (NH_4^+) ions (see Fig. 3.20). Although the liver is capable of metabolizing NH_4^+ to urea, it is only by secretion of NH_4^+ in the kidney that HCO_3^- can be regenerated to serve as a buffer in the plasma. However, 50% of NH_4^+ secreted into the proximal tubule is reabsorbed by the thick ascending limb of the loop of Henle and accumulates in the cells of the medullary interstitium (see Fig. 3.21). Fig. 3.20 illustrates the secretion and handling of ammonia,

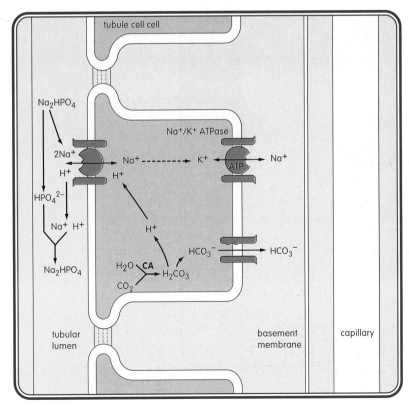

Fig. 3.19 Conversion of alkaline phosphate to acid phosphate in the tubule lumen. Conversion of alkaline phosphate to acid phosphate liberates free sodium. This is transported into the tubule cell by an Na^+/H^+ antiporter, causing H^+ secretion into the lumen and increased HCO_3^- reabsorption by the tubule cells. (CA, carbonic anhydrase.)

53

while Fig. 3.21 shows NH_3 and NH_4^+ handling by the nephrons.

Acidosis results in increased NH_4^+ excretion because:

- Acidosis stimulates enzymes that deaminate glutamine.
- Increased H^+ secretion results in NH_3 production, which in turn results in increased NH_4^+ in the collecting tubules. The conversion of NH_3 to NH_4^+ maintains a gradient for NH_3 secretion. Therefore, increased NH_3 /NH_4^+ is removed from the medulla.

Acid–base disturbances

There are four main types:

- Respiratory acidosis.
- Respiratory alkalosis.
- Metabolic (non-respiratory origin) acidosis.
- Metabolic alkalosis.

Metabolic disturbances result from changes in cellular metabolism or diet, and not pCO_2. A change in the body fluid pH causes the buffering system to become effective. As a result, there may be very little change in arterial pH despite acid–base imbalance. A change in the arterial pH reflects a change in the pH of body cells.

The Davenport diagram is a graph of the plasma HCO_3^- versus plasma pH. It is useful in diagnosing acid–base disturbances (see Fig. 3.22):

Compensation and correction

Compensation is the restoration of normal pH even though the acid–base imbalance is still present. Correction is the restoration of both the pH and acid–base imbalance to normal:

$$H_2O + CO_2 \leftrightarrow H_2CO_3 \leftrightarrow H^+ + HCO_3^-$$
$$pH \propto [HCO_3^-]/pCO_2$$

Therefore if two variables (e.g. pH and pCO_2) are known, $[HCO_3^-]$ can be calculated.

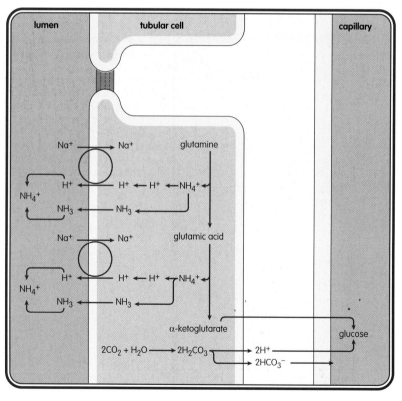

Fig. 3.20 Secretion and handling of NH_3.

By using the arterial blood gas results, an acid–base imbalance can be diagnosed. For example, if pH = 7.2 and pCO_2 is 9.3 kPa, by looking at the graph, it can be seen that HCO_3^- will be increased. This is a respiratory acidosis.

Examples of acid–base disturbances
Respiratory acidosis
The causes of respiratory acidosis are:
- Chronic bronchitis.
- Emphysema.
- Obstruction of the airway (e.g. tumour, foreign body).
- Mechanical chest injuries.
- Asthma.
- Drugs—general anaesthetic, morphine, barbiturates (respiratory centre depressant).
- Injuries and infections to the respiratory centre in the brain stem.

Arterial blood gases (ABG) show pCO_2 over 6.0 kPa and decreased pH. Clinically the respiratory system cannot remove enough CO_2, resulting in an increased CO_2 and increased pCO_2. Therefore the following equation is shifted to the right:

$$CO_2 + H_2O \xrightarrow{} H_2CO_3 \xrightarrow{} H^+ + HCO_3^-$$

This results in increased H^+ and increased HCO_3^-. The increased H^+ results in increased H^+ secretion and increased HCO_3^- reabsorption. This restores pH and constitutes a compensatory response. The acid–base disturbance is not corrected, because the pCO_2 and $[HCO_3^-]$ are still high. Correction would require a respiratory effort to decrease pCO_2.

Fig. 3.22 illustrates acid–base disturbances with compensatory changes demonstrated on the Davenport diagram.

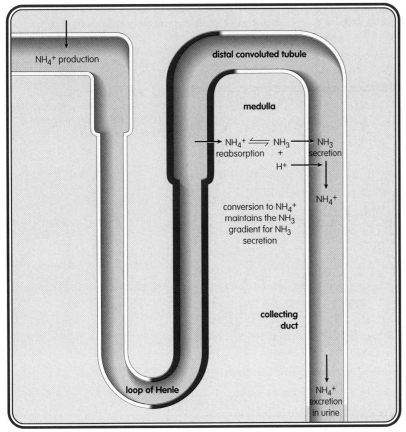

Fig. 3.21 Handling of NH_3 and NH_4^+ by nephrons.

NH_4^+ production

distal convoluted tubule

medulla

$NH_4^+ \rightleftharpoons NH_3$ reabsorption $+$ NH_3 secretion

H^+

NH_4^+

conversion to NH_4^+ maintains the NH_3 gradient for NH_3 secretion

collecting duct

loop of Henle

NH_4^+ excretion in urine

Respiratory alkalosis

The causes of respiratory alkalosis are:
- Decreased pO_2, which triggers chemoreceptors in the carotid body, resulting in hyperventilation and decreased pCO_2.
- High altitude.
- Fever.
- Brain stem damage resulting in hyperventilation.
- Hysterical overbreathing.

The ABG results show a pCO_2 of less than 4.7 kPa. Clinically too much CO_2 is removed by the respiratory system. Therefore the following equation is shifted to the left:

$$CO_2 + H_2O \overset{\longleftarrow}{\longleftrightarrow} H_2CO_3 \overset{\longleftarrow}{\longleftrightarrow} H^+ + HCO_3^-$$

This results in decreased [H$^+$], and hence an increased pH and a slight decrease in [HCO$_3^-$]. The compensatory response is decreased H$^+$ secretion, increased HCO$_3^-$ excretion and decreased HCO$_3^-$ reabsorption, thus restoring pH. Correction would require rectification of the respiratory defect that results in decreased ventilation (see Fig. 3.22).

Metabolic acidosis

The causes of metabolic acidosis are:
- Ingestion of acids (H$^+$).
- Excess metabolic production of H$^+$ (e.g. lactate acidosis, diabetic ketoacidosis).
- Loss of HCO$_3^-$ (e.g. severe diarrhoea, drainage from fistulae).
- Renal disease.

ABG results show a normal pCO_2 and decreased pH. There is an increase in [H$^+$]. Therefore, the following equation is shifted to the left:

$$CO_2 + H_2O \overset{\longleftarrow}{\longleftrightarrow} H_2CO_3 \overset{\longleftarrow}{\longleftrightarrow} H^+ + HCO_3^-$$

As a result, there is a decreased [HCO$_3^-$].

The decreased pH stimulates peripheral chemoreceptors and stimulates respiration to cause hyperventilation. This respiratory compensation decreases pCO_2 and returns the pH to normal, although HCO$_3^-$ falls further. The fall in HCO$_3^-$ hinders the corrective response of the kidneys, which is to increase HCO$_3^-$ reabsorption and production of titratable acid.

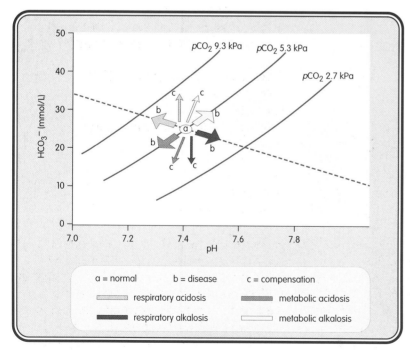

Fig. 3.22 Acid and base disturbances with compensatory changes demonstrated on the Davenport diagram.

a = normal   b = disease   c = compensation

respiratory acidosis ▭   metabolic acidosis ▬

respiratory alkalosis ▬   metabolic alkalosis ▭

The anion gap helps in the diagnosis of metabolic acidosis. This represents the difference between anions and cations and represents unestimated anions (e.g. phosphates, ketones, lactate):

$$\text{Anion gap} = ([K^+] + [Na^+]) - ([Cl^-] + [HCO_3^-])$$

The normal range is 8–16 mmol/L.

Metabolic alkalosis
The causes of metabolic alkalosis are:
- Loss of acid (e.g. vomiting).
- Ingestion of alkali.

ABG results show a normal pCO_2 and increased pH is decreased by combination of H^+ with base. Therefore, the following equation is shifted to the right

$$CO_2 + H_2O \longleftrightarrow H_2CO_3 \longleftrightarrow H^+ + HCO_3^-$$

$$H^+ + OH^- \rightarrow H_2O$$

HCO_3^- is increased.

Respiratory compensation occurs. The decreased H^+ (increased pH) acts on chemoreceptors, resulting in decreased ventilation and increased pCO_2, therefore driving the equation to the right and returning the pH to normal, but further increasing HCO_3^-. This hampers correction (see Fig. 3.22).

Fig. 3.23 summarizes acid–base disturbances.

Summary of acid–base disturbances			
Acid–base disturbance	**pH**	**PCO$_2$**	**HCO$_3^-$**
respiratory acidosis	↓	↑	↑
respiratory alkalosis	↑	↓	↓
metabolic acidosis	↓	normal	↓
metabolic alkalosis	↑	normal	↑

Fig. 3.23 Summary of acid–base disturbances (uncompensated).

REGULATION OF POTASSIUM, CALCIUM, MAGNESIUM, AND PHOSPHATE

Potassium (K⁺)
K^+ is the main intracellular cation. Its concentration is very important in the function of excitable tissues (e.g. nerves and muscles). Intracellular and extracellular K^+ concentration determines the resting potentials of these tissues. Therefore K^+ concentration is important for survival. Concentration is as follows:
- Total body K^+: 3–4 mmol/L.
- Intracellular fluid (ICF) K^+: 98%; 150–160 mmol/L.
- Extracellular fluid (ECF) K^+: 2%; 4–5 mmol/L.

Clinical features and causes of K⁺ disturbances
Hypokalaemia
Causes of a decreased K^+ concentration are:
- Vomiting.
- Diarrhoea.
- Diuretics.
- Excess insulin.
- Renal tubular acidosis.

Hypokalaemia is symptomless until K^+ concentration falls below 2–2.5 mmol/L. The low K^+ concentration results in a decreased resting potential (more negative) (i.e. hyperpolarization of nerve and muscle cells meaning that cells are less sensitive to depolarizing stimuli and therefore less excitable). This results in a decreased number of action potentials and paralysis.

- **What is the normal pH range and explain why and how it is tightly controlled.**
- **Discuss the role of kidney in regulating acid–base balance.**
- **Explain the four acid–base disturbances discussing their causes, their arterial blood gas pictures, and their clinical pictures. Use the Davenport diagram as a reference.**

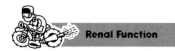

The effects of hypokalaemia are:
- Muscle weakening, which starts in the lower extremities and progresses upwards (death is usually by paralysis of respiratory muscles).
- Impaired liver conversion of glucose to glycogen.
- Vasoconstriction.
- Impaired ADH action, causing thirst and polyuria and no concentration of urine.
- Metabolic alkalosis due to an increase in intracellular H^+ concentration.

Treatment involves treating the underlying cause, and careful administration of potassium salt (oral or intravenously) may be required.

Hyperkalaemia
Causes of an increased K^+ concentration are:
- Ingestion of K^+.
- Metabolic acidosis.
- Insulin deficiency.
- Excess cell breakdown (e.g. after cytotoxic treatment).
- Renal failure.

Hyperkalaemia is symptomless. The increased K^+ concentration results in cell depolarization and increased excitability. The resting potential may be above the threshold potential, so cells cannot repolarize after an action potential, leading to paralysis. Death results from cardiac arrest due to arrhythmias (broad complex ECG) when the K^+ concentration is >7 mmol/L.

Treatment may involve:
- Dextrose and insulin to drive K^+ into cells.
- HCO_3^- to correct acidosis to drive K^+ into cells.
- Calcium salts to protect excitable tissues (of heart) against toxic effects of K^+.
- K^+ removal from body using loop diuretics, exchange resins (i.e. calcium resonium), and dialysis.

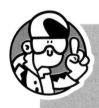

Hypokalaemia and hyperkalaemia are life-threatening because of adverse effects on excitable tissues.

Kidney's transport of K^+
K^+ is freely filtered in the glomerulus. In the proximal tubule 80–90% is reabsorbed:
- Passively.
- Through tight junctions (paracellular).
- Via a concentration gradient.

In the distal tubule:
- K^+ reabsorption and leakage back are similar in the early distal tubule.
- The late distal tubule and collecting ducts secrete K^+ (passively via an electrochemical gradient) depending upon the body's needs—increased cellular K^+ concentration results in increased secretion and vice versa.

Changes in the distal tubular lumen also influence the rate of K^+ secretion. Fig. 3.24 illustrates transportation of K^+ in the kidney.

ADH stimulates the secretion of K^+ by the collecting ducts by enhancing Na^+ reabsorption. Aldosterone increases K^+ secretion. Increased plasma K^+ concentration results in increased aldosterone production by the adrenal cortex and therefore an increased plasma aldosterone concentration, which in turn increases K^+ secretion and therefore K^+ excretion.

Calcium (Ca^{2+})
Ca^{2+} is present mainly in bone and has an important extraskeletal function. The threshold potential of cell membranes of nerve and muscle for action potentials varies inversely with plasma calcium concentration. Thus it is important to maintain calcium levels.

There are two types of calcium concentration in the plasma:
- Ionized Ca^{2+}, which is physiologically important (1.25 mmol/L).
- Ca^{2+} bound to protein—mainly albumin (1.25 mmol/L).

Ca^{2+} concentrations are as follows:
- Total Ca^{2+}—2.50 mmol/L.
- Interstitial fluid total Ca^{2+}—1.25 mmol/L.
- Intracellular Ca^{2+}—0.0001 mmol/L; found in smooth endothelial reticulum and mitochondria, complexed with calmodulin.
- ECF Ca^{2+}—1.25 mmol/L.

It is important to maintain a low intracellular Ca^{2+}.

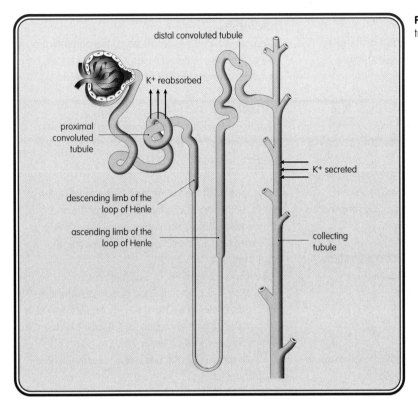

Fig. 3.24 Summary of potassium transportation in the kidney.

Clinical features and causes of Ca^{2+} disturbances

Hypocalcaemia

Decreased Ca^{2+} results in tetany with convulsions, hand and feet muscle paralysis, and cardiac arrhythmias. Causes are:

- Hypoparathyroidism.
- Rickets and osteomalacia (low vitamin D).
- Hypomagnesaemia.
- Pancreatitis.
- Alkalosis when there is decreased H^+ to bind to protein so more Ca^{2+} can bind; this results in decreased ionized Ca^{2+} yet total Ca^{2+} is unchanged. Alkalosis occurs in patients with chronic renal failure because of hyperphosphataemia (the Ca^{2+} and PO_4^{3-} product is constant) and low levels of activated vitamin D.

Hypercalcaemia

Causes of hypercalcaemia are:

- Primary hyperparathyroidism.
- Sudden acidosis resulting in conversion of bound calcium to ionized Ca^{2+}.
- Increased intestinal absorption due to excess vitamin D or ingestion of calcium (milk–alkali syndrome).
- Bone destruction resulting in increased Ca^{2+} release from bone—usually due to secondary deposits from malignancy or myeloma.
- Production of tumour-associated humoral hypercalcaemic agents.
- Granulomatous disease (sarcoid).
- Drugs—thiazides.
- Tertiary hyperparathyroidism in chronic renal failure.
- Increase in magnesium.

Symptoms of hypercalcaemia are:

- Renal calculi.
- Behaviour disturbance (because of effects on higher cerebral functions).
- Constipation due to decreased intestinal mobility.
- Renal damage.
- Calcification outside the skeletal system.
- Polyuria.
- Polydipsia.

Kidney's transport of Ca^{2+}

Only ionized Ca^{2+} is filtered through the glomerulus (approximately 50% plasma Ca^{2+}). Reabsorption proceeds in the following way:

- In the proximal tubule 70% is reabsorbed by diffusion, Ca^{2+}-activated ATPase, and Ca^{2+}/Na^+ countertransport system.
- In the thick ascending loop of Henle 20–25% is reabsorbed passively.
- In the distal convoluted tubule 5–10% is reabsorbed against an electrochemical gradient.
- In the collecting tubule less than 0.5% is reabsorbed against an electrochemical gradient.

Calcium and phosphate homoeostasis

Ca^{2+} and PO_4^{3-} concentrations are inversely proportional.

$$[Ca^{2+}] \times [PO_4^{3-}] = constant$$

Therefore, any increase in Ca^{2+} results in a decrease in PO_4^{3-} whereas a decreased Ca^{2+} results in an increased PO_4^{3-} concentration.

Ca^{2+} and PO_4^{3-} enter the ECF via the intestine (diet) and bone stores. They leave the ECF via the kidneys (urine) and move into the bone.

Regulation of Ca^{2+} and PO_4^{3-} is effected by parathyroid hormone (PTH), vitamin D, and calcitonin.

Parathyroid hormone (PTH)

PTH is a polypeptide secreted by the parathyroid gland. Decreased Ca^{2+} results in PTH release and increased Ca^{2+} results in the suppression of PTH release. PO_4^{3-} also affects PTH release, both directly and secondary to reciprocal changes in Ca^{2+}. Fig. 3.25 illustrates mechanisms of Ca^{2+} and PO_4^{3-} homoeostasis. Vitamin D may also affect PTH release as it alters sensitivity of the gland to Ca^{2+}.

Vitamin D

Vitamin D refers to a group of closely related sterols obtained from the diet or by the action of ultraviolet light on certain provitamins. It is metabolized to 1,25-dihydroxycholecalciferol by the liver and kidney. This causes an increase in Ca^{2+} and PO_4^{3-} by:

- Enhancing intestinal absorption of Ca^{2+}.
- Increasing Ca^{2+} release from bone.
- Decreasing Ca^{2+} and PO_4^{3-} excretion.

Calcitonin

Calcitonin is a peptide produced by the parafollicular cells of the thyroid. It decreases Ca^{2+} release from bone causing a decrease in ECF Ca^{2+} concentration.

Phosphate

Phosphate is present in the plasma and interstitial fluid as:

- 'Acid' phosphate $H_2PO_4^-$.
- 'Alkaline' phosphate HPO_4^{3-}.

The proportion of the two forms is determined by the pH. In cells, both inorganic forms (acid phosphate and alkaline phosphate) and organic forms (ATP, ADP, and cAMP) are found. Plasma phosphate concentration is 0.8–1.3 mmol/L.

Renal handling of PO_4^{3-} is as follows:

- Alkaline phosphate and acid phosphate are filtered by the glomerulus in a ratio of 4:1. Alkaline phosphate is converted to acid phosphate in the tubule as a result of H^+ secretion (Fig. 3.19).
- Most filtered PO_4^{3-} (95%) is reabsorbed in the early proximal tubule.
- Renal PO_4^{3-} excretion is increased by PTH.

Magnesium (Mg^{2+})

Magnesium is an intracellular cation that:

- Controls mitochondrial oxidative metabolism and so regulates energy production.
- Is vital for protein synthesis.
- Regulates K^+ and Ca^{2+} channels in cell membranes.

Its plasma concentration is 2.12–2.65 mmol/L. About 20% is protein bound. Total body magnesium is 28 g of which:

- 55% is in bone.
- 44% is in ICF.
- 4–25% is in plasma.
- 0.6% is in ECF.

Clinical features and causes of Mg^{2+} disturbances

Hypomagnesaemia

Clinical features are non-specific. Causes are:

- Decreased intake.
- Diarrhoea.
- Absorption disorder including fat absorption defects.
- Renal wasting—intrinsic (Bartter's syndrome), extrinsic (diuretics—thiazides).

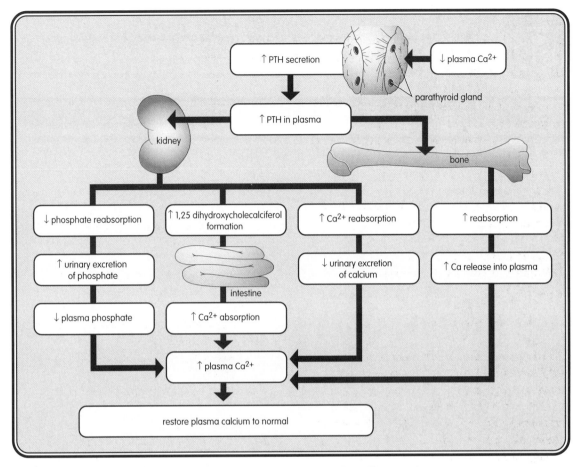

Fig. 3.25 Mechanisms of Ca^{2+} and phosphate homoeostasis. (PTH, parathyroid hormone.)

Decreased Mg^{2+} results in a decreased Ca^{2+}, but the mechanism is unexplained.

Renal handling of Mg^{2+}

This is as follows:
- In the glomerulus ionized Mg (75%) is filtered.
- In the proximal tubule there is some reabsorption (15%).
- In the thick ascending loop of Henle 60% is reabsorbed—the $Na^+/K^+/Cl^-$ co-transporter system causes a lumen-positive potential causing Mg^{2+} absorption through the paracellular route. A Na^+/Mg^{2+} antiport and Mg^{2+} ATPase transport system also exists.

- In the distal convoluted tubule 2–5% is reabsorbed.
- In the collecting tubule 0.5% is reabsorbed.

Regulation

T_m for absorption is equal to the concentration of Mg^{2+} filtered. Therefore an increase in Mg^{2+} results in increased filtering, which therefore exceeds the T_m, resulting in increased excretion.

There is intrinsic regulation by cells of the thick ascending loop of Henle—if Mg^{2+} decreases, cell transport of Mg^{2+} increases.

PTH increases reabsorption of Mg^{2+} in the thick ascending loop of Henle.

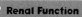

For potassium, calcium, magnesium, and phosphate, discuss the following:
- Their importance in the body.
- Their concentration.
- How the kidney transports them.
- High and low concentrations.

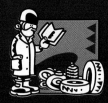

4. Renal Function in Disease

SYSTEMIC DISEASES THAT AFFECT RENAL FUNCTION

Congestive cardiac failure (CCF)

CCF occurs as a result of an imbalance between the function of the heart as a pump and its work load (i.e. providing the body with its metabolic requirements); a normal heart may fail under high loads, but an abnormal heart will fail under normal loads. This results in hypoperfusion of tissues and sodium and water retention. CCF is the main complication of all types of severe heart disease.

One of the most important consequences of a decrease in cardiac output (CO) is renal hypoperfusion. The kidney senses this as a sign of effective hypovolaemia and the kidney retains NaCl and water as a compensatory mechanism to increase the circulating volume (Fig. 4.1). As the kidney attempts to increase the circulating fluid volume there is oedema formation. If there is fluid transudation from the capillaries in the lungs as a result of an abrupt rise in pulmonary venous pressure, pulmonary oedema may result.

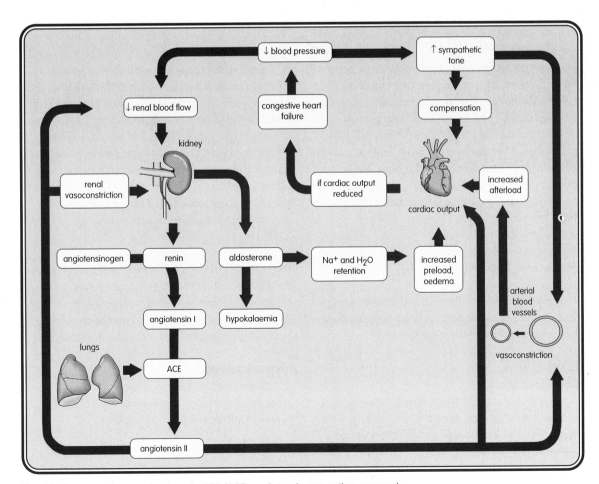

Fig. 4.1 Compensatory mechanisms in CCF. (ACE, angiotensin-converting enzyme.)

Treatment and management

The management of such conditions consists of reducing the fluid load within the body and thereby decreasing the workload of the heart:

- Symptomatic relief from pulmonary oedema can be achieved with diuretics.
- Preload reduction is achieved by venodilatation with nitrates.
- Afterload can be reduced using vasodilators such as hydralazine.
- ACE inhibitors are also an important drug in the treatment of CCF since they counteract the compensatory mechanisms of the heart by reducing the effect of angiotensin II and the fluid-retaining effect of aldosterone.

For further information refer to *Crash Course: Cardiovascular System*.

Hypovolaemia and shock

Shock is a life-threatening state in which there is widespread hypoperfusion of the tissues as a result of either an inadequate circulating blood volume or pump failure. Since not enough oxygen and nutrients are delivered to the cells, the resulting hypoxic state within the cells causes a shift from aerobic to anaerobic metabolism and there is inefficient clearance of the metabolites, which build up in the cell. Hypovolaemia and mild shock cause tiredness, dizziness, and a feeling of thirst. A severe decrease in the circulating volume will stimulate sympathetic activity to maintain the blood pressure (BP) by:

- Tachycardia.
- Peripheral vasoconstriction.
- Increase in myocardial contractility.

If compensatory mechanisms are insufficient, tissue hypoxia and necrosis may occur in vulnerable organs (e.g. acute tubular necrosis in the kidneys).

Types of shock

Cardiogenic shock

This occurs as a result of sudden pump failure from ischaemic heart disease, arrhythmias, or outflow obstruction, causing a sudden decrease in cardiac output. As a result, tissue perfusion decreases dramatically. Venous pressure increases, causing pulmonary or peripheral oedema.

Hypovolaemic shock

Hypovolaemic shock result from:

- Exogenous losses of plasma (e.g. due to burns), of whole blood (e.g. due to haemorrhage), or of water and electrolytes (e.g. due to diarrhoea and vomiting).
- Endogenous losses of fluid (e.g. due to sepsis and anaphylaxis).

Fig. 4.2 shows the response to a fall in circulating fluid volume. Sympathetic vasoconstrictive activity spares the arterioles of the cerebral cortex. To ensure that excessive vasoconstriction is avoided in the kidneys there is an increase in the secretion of vasodilating prostaglandins (PGE_2 and PGI_2) within the kidneys stimulated by arteriolar vasoconstriction. In this way an adequate blood flow is maintained through the kidney to allow sufficient glomerular filtration unless the shock is severe. The loss of large amounts of fluid has two major consequences:

- Volume depletion (decreases tissue perfusion).
- Electrolyte and acid–base disturbance.

Since Na^+ is involved in the co-transport of H^+, K^+, and Cl^- there is a disturbance in acid–base balance as a result of excessive Na^+ reabsorption. Cl^- is reabsorbed in equal quantities, but there is increased secretion of H^+ and K^+ resulting in metabolic alkalosis (contraction alkalosis) and hypokalaemia. This tendency to alkalosis is balanced by the shift to anaerobic metabolism as a result of hypoxia in the tissues. A severe metabolic acidosis will occur when the ability of the tubular cells to secrete H^+ is exceeded by the acid production of the cells as a result of anaerobic respiration.

Treatment

The treatment for such a metabolic acidosis consists in the administration of fluids, blood, or plasma as appropriate to restore the extracellular volume. HCO_3^- is required only if there there is severe acidosis (pH less than 7.2) (see Chapter 3 for acid–base disturbances).

Hypertension

BP is determined by the interaction of genetic and environmental factors, which regulate CO and total peripheral resistance (TPR). For example:

$$BP = CO \times TPR$$

The kidneys contribute to BP control by regulating ECF volume. They also release vasoactive substances:

- Vasoconstrictors—angiotensin II.
- Vasodilators—prostaglandins.

Renal autoregulation maintains renal function in the face of wide variations in systolic BP. Any change in the ECF will affect the BP. By controlling water and sodium excretion, the kidney can help compensate for any changes in ECF. A disturbance in these regulatory mechanisms will cause hypertension. Hypertension, as defined by the World Health Organization (WHO) is a sustained BP higher than 160/90 mmHg.

Essential hypertension

This accounts for about 90% of all causes of hypertension and the cause is unknown. In the initial stages there is an increase in cardiac output and this is thought to be related to sympathetic overactivity. In the later stages the increase in BP is maintained by an increase in the TPR, but cardiac output is normal. Hypertensive changes seen in the kidney include:

- Arteriosclerosis of the major renal arteries.
- Hyalinization of the small vessels with intimal thickening.

This may lead to chronic renal damage (hypertensive nephrosclerosis) and a reduction in the size of the kidneys.

A rare and rapidly progressing form of hypertension is known as accelerated hypertension, or malignant hypertension. This is characterized by fibrinoid necrosis of the vessel wall, and ischaemic damage to the brain and kidney may result, leading to a high mortality if left untreated.

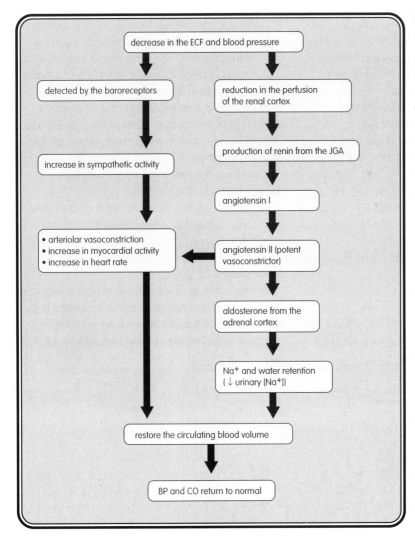

Fig. 4.2 Response to a fall in circulating fluid volume. (BP, blood pressure; CO, cardiac output; ECF, extracellular fluid; JGA, juxtaglomerular apparatus.)

Secondary hypertension

A cause of hypertension is discovered in less than 10% of hypertensive patients. Secondary causes include renal (80%), endocrine, and cardiovascular causes, pregnancy, and drugs.

Renal mechanisms causing hypertension include:
- Impaired sodium and water excretion, increasing blood volume.
- Stimulation of the renin–angiotensin–aldosterone system.

Renal artery stenosis

There are two types:
- Atherosclerosis—common.
- Fibromuscular dysplasia—rare (seen in young women) (see Fig. 9.11).

The effect of a narrowed renal vessel is to decrease the pressure in the afferent arterioles, which stimulates the juxtaglomerular apparatus to secrete reninThis results in an increased plasma level of angiotensin II which causes vasoconstriction and release of aldosterone. Aldosterone promotes fluid retention

Transluminal angioplasty is used to dilate the stenotic region. Reconstructive vascular surgery or nephrectomy are other options. With these interventions up to 50% of the patients are cured or improved.

Intrinsic renal diseases

These include chronic glomerulonephritis (GN), chronic pyelonephritis, and polycystic kidney disease.

Primary glomerular disease presents with hypertension earlier and is more severe than in patients with renal interstitial disease.

Endocrine causes

The endocrine causes are:
- Cushing's syndrome.

- Oestrogen (i.e. the contraceptive pill and pregnancy).
- Phaeochromocytoma (rare).
- Primary hyperaldosteronism.

Primary hyperaldosteronism is a rare condition in which an adrenal cortical adenoma increases the secretion of aldosterone (Conn's syndrome) (Fig. 4.3). Patients present with hypertension and hypokalaemia. Diagnosis is made with a triad of:
- Hypokalaemia.
- Increased aldosterone.
- Decreased renin.

It is unknown why the result is hypertension since the volume expansion is small. Treatment is by surgical removal of the adenoma, with a cure rate of 60%.

Management of hypertension

The detection and management of hypertension can be difficult since it presents asymptomatically and many patients are reluctant to take medication if they feel well. It is very important to rule out any of the secondary causes of hypertension.

Hypertension is an important cause of strokes, cardiac failure, myocardial infarction, and renal failure. Effective treatment will improve the prognosis for each of these conditions.

General measures include weight reduction, decrease of heavy alcohol intake, salt restriction, regular exercise. Many different drugs are used in the treatment of hypertension and these will be discussed later in this chapter..

Liver disease

Patients with liver disease and especially those with portal vein hypertension and ascites may have a reduced urine flow (oliguria). It is thought that nitric oxide (NO) causes peripheral vasodilatation and venous pooling, resulting in

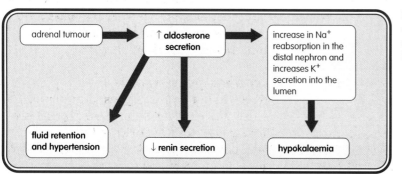

Fig. 4.3 Mechanism by which an adrenal tumour (Conn's syndrome) causes secondary hypertension.

the activation of the renin–angiotensin–aldosterone system. Sodium and water retention results from the apparent decrease in arterial blood volume. The increase in the hydrostatic pressure of the portal vein, as a result of increased resistance in the liver due to hepatic cirrhosis, causes an accumulation of fluid in the peritoneal cavity (ascites) as fluid is forced out of the interstitial capillaries. The transudation of fluid out of the capillaries results in a further decrease in circulating blood volume, which once again stimulates the renin–angiotensin–aldosterone system. This results in a positive feedback loop promoting hypertension.

Liver disease may also affect the synthesis of albumin. This decreases the oncotic (colloid osmotic) pressure in the capillaries, favouring fluid movement out and worsening the ascites, and further decreasing circulating blood volume.

Nephrotic syndrome

This syndrome is characterized by:
- Proteinuria.
- Hypoalbuminaemia.
- Oedema.
- Secondary hypercholesterolaemia.

The permeability of the glomerular filter to albumin increases as a result of damage to the glomerular basement membrane and increase in pore size. In an adult a loss of more than 3–5 g of albumin per day will cause hypoalbuminaemia. Filtered protein can be reabsorbed by endocytosis, but the capacity of this system is limited and readily exceeded, when protein loss in the urine will result. The albumin content within the capillary is very important in maintaining the colloid osmotic pressure. If this is reduced the forces favouring fluid movement back into the capillaries decrease, causing oedema in the peripheral tissues. The decreased circulating volume activates the renin–angiotensin–aldosterone sytem leading to further sodium and water retention, with resultant oedema.

Treatment

Management includes:
- General measures, such as dietary sodium restriction and a thiazide diuretic.
- Specific measures and treatment of underlying causes, e.g. in minimal change disease, high-dose corticosteroid therapy will treat protein leakage in 90% of children. The response in adults is much lower.

Diabetes mellitus

Nodular and diffuse glomerulosclerosis, arteriolar lesions, and exudative lesions such as the fibrin cap are all renal histological manifestations of diabetes mellitus. Pyelonephritis is a common complication and can result in renal papillary necrosis.

Diabetic nephropathy is often clinically manifest as the nephrotic syndrome. Characteristic histological changes include an increase in the mesangial matrix with two morphological patterns:
- Nodular glomerulosclerosis (Kimmelstiel–Wilson nodules—nodular accumulations of mesangial matrix material).
- Diffuse glomerulosclerosis—diffusely increased areas of mesangial matrix.

On electron microscopy there is an increase in the thickness of the glomerular basement membrane.

Chronic renal damage due to diabetes is associated with, and is accelerated by, hypertension. The commonest reason for needing dialysis in developed countries is CRF due to diabetes mellitus.

Immune disorders affecting the kidney

Systemic lupus erythematosus (SLE)

SLE affects women (70–80% of cases) more than men. It is characterized by the presence of antinuclear antibodies and widespread immune complex-mediated inflammatory lesions in many organs. The renal lesions are the most important clinically and are the major prognostic factor in the outcome of the disease. Glomerular changes vary from minimal involvement to diffuse proliferative disease with:
- Mesangial immune complex deposition.
- Thickening of the basement membrane.
- Endothelial proliferation.

Subendothelial deposition of immune complexes are diagnostic and these produce a characteristic wire-loop appearance seen by light microscopy. Patients present with hypertension and oedema. SLE is frequently a progressive condition leading to CRF.

Wegener's granulomatosis

Wegener's granulomatosis is a vasculitis syndrome with an unknown aetiology. It is characterized by necrotizing granulomatous vasculitis of the blood vessels in the kidney and other organs. Clinically patients present with necrotizing glomerulonephritis.

Infections

Poststreptococcal glomerulonephritis

This disorder most often follows or accompanies infection with nephritogenic strains of group A β-haemolytic streptococci. It is followed by complete recovery in almost all children and most adults. Glomerulonephritis is the result of immune complex disease due to antigen–antibody complexes of streptococcal origin. Laboratory abnormalities associated with the infection include urinary red cells and red cell casts, increased serum creatinine and urea, decreased plasma C3, and an increased titre of antistreptolysin O (ASO).

Bacterial endocarditis

Bacterial endocarditis can also be complicated by immune complex disease. A focal GN is occasionally seen following infection of the endocardium. This may cause microscopic haematuria, fluid retention and renal impairment.

- Explain the compensatory mechanisms that come into effect in CCF.
- Outline the different types of shock and their consequences for renal physiology.
- Define hypertension; state the two main types and outline the causes of hypertension.
- Describe how the kidney may be affected by diabetes mellitus.
- Which immune disorders have manifestations in the kidney?

INTERVENTIONS IN RENAL DISEASE

Control of fluid balance

Diuretics

Diuresis means to increase the volume of urine. Diuretics are used in medicine to increase the amount of urine by increasing renal sodium excretion (natriuresis), which is passively followed by water elimination. Diuretics act on specific anatomical sites of the nephron (Fig. 4.4). Each type of diuretic has specific actions on the normal physiology of a particular segment. Diuretics:

- Act on the membrane transport proteins found on the luminal surface.
- Interfere with hormone receptors.
- Inhibit enzyme activity.

Osmotic diuretics

Osmotic diuresis can be induced by a substance that is not reabsorbed in the tubule. The proximal tubule and the descending limb of the loop of Henle allow free movement of water molecules. If an agent such as mannitol is introduced into the tubular fluid, it is not absorbed and is osmotically active. Thus water is retained, promoting water diuresis. As a result of the increased urine flow the time of contact between the tubular fluid and cells is reduced and so less sodium is reabsorbed.

Osmotic diuretics are used to increase urine volume when renal haemodynamics are compromised and thus prevent anuria. They are also used to reduce intracranial pressures in neurological conditions and intraocular pressures before ophthalmic surgery.

Excessive use without adequate fluid replacement may cause dehydration and hypernatraemia.

Potassium-sparing diuretics

Potassium-sparing diuretics antagonize the effect of aldosterone:

- In the collecting ducts (e.g. spironolactone).
- By inhibiting the uptake of Na^+ in the cells of the distal nephron (e.g. amiloride and triamterene).

Aldosterone increases the activity of the Na^+/K^+ ATPase, potassium, and sodium channels, resulting in Na^+ absorption and K^+ secretion.

Spironolactone (a mineralcorticoid analogue) competes with aldosterone for the receptor site. This reduces sodium reabsorption in the distal nephron and decreases K+ secretion (potassium sparing activity).

Potassium-sparing diuretics are fairly weak and are often used in combination with loop diuretics or thiazides to prevent K+ loss.

These diuretics are used in cases of mineralocorticoid excess such as primary aldosteronism (Conn's syndrome) or ectopic ACTH production. They may also be useful in secondary aldosteronism where salt and water retention have occurred (e.g. CCF, nephrotic syndrome, liver disease, and hypovolaemia).

The side effects of potassium-sparing diuretics include:
- Hyperkalaemia—which can be mild to life-threatening and results from an increase in H+ retention as a result of reduced Na+ absorption; oral K+ supplements should be stopped.
- Endocrine effects with spironolactone (e.g. gynaecomastia).

Potassium-sparing diuretics are contraindicated in patients with chronic renal insufficiency.

Loop diuretics

These agents prevent extrusion of sodium from the thick ascending limb of the loop of Henle into medullary interstitium. Examples include:
- Frusemide.
- Bumetanide.
- Piretanide.

Loop diuretics act by inhibiting the Na+/K+/2Cl− co-transporter on the luminal membrane of the cells. This causes a decrease in Na+ reabsorption and dilution of the osmotic gradient in the medulla, resulting in an increase in water and Na+ excretion (up to 30% of the filtered sodium can be excreted with high doses of the drugs). The decrease in the positive lumen potential due to the retention of cations causes an increase in Ca^{2+} and Mg^{2+} excretion. As a result of the faster rate of flow of the diluted tubular fluid in the distal tubule there is increased K+ secretion and therefore loop diuretics can be used in the management of hyperkalaemia to reduce total body K+ stores.

The most important uses of loop diuretics are for:
- Acute pulmonary oedema.
- Acute hypercalcaemia.

Frusemide reduces end-diastolic ventricular filling pressure, relieves pulmonary congestion, and reduces peripheral oedema. Loop diuretics can also be used in acute renal failure to increase urine output and encourage K+ excretion.

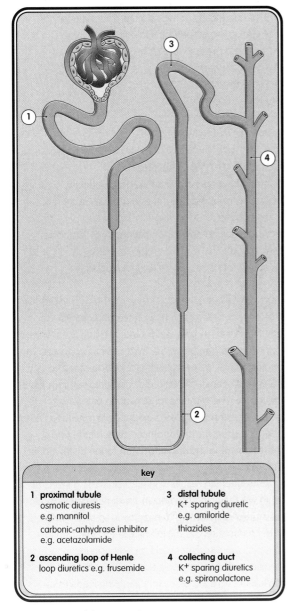

key

1	**proximal tubule**	3	**distal tubule**
	osmotic diuresis e.g. mannitol		K+ sparing diuretic e.g. amiloride
	carbonic-anhydrase inhibitor e.g. acetazolamide		thiazides
2	**ascending loop of Henle** loop diuretics e.g. frusemide	4	**collecting duct** K+ sparing diuretics e.g. spironolactone

Fig. 4.4 Sites of diuretic action.

The side effects of loop diuretics include:

- Hypokalaemic metabolic alkalosis.
- Ototoxicity (dose-related reversible auditory loss).
- Hyperuricaemia (can precipitate attacks of gout).
- Hypomagnesaemia.
- Allergic reactions.

Side effects of thiazide diuretics: HyperGLUC (hyper glucose, lipid, uric acid, and calcium).

Carbonic anhydrase (CA) inhibitors

CA is found in many places in the nephron. The principal site is the brush border of the luminal membrane of the proximal tubule cells. CA catalyses the dehydration of H_2CO_3 to H_2O and CO_2 within the tubular lumen. This reaction is driven by secretion of H^+ into the lumen, by co-transport with Na^+:

$$H^+ + HCO_3^- \leftrightarrow H_2CO_3 \leftrightarrow H_2O + CO_2$$

Once in the cell, H_2CO_3 is reformed under the influence of CA in the cell, the HCO_3^- ions are reabsorbed, and H^+ is secreted back into the lumen (see Fig. 2.23).

CA inhibitors interfere with the action of carbonic anhydrase and inhibit HCO_3^- reabsorption. The highest dose of the CA inhibitor, acetazolamide, can inhibit up to 85% of the resorptive capacity of HCO_3^- in the proximal tubule. The presence of HCO_3^- in the lumen reduces Na^+ reabsorption, which continues into the distal nephron where it enhances K^+ secretion.

CA inhibitors are weak diuretics capable of causing the excretion of only about 5–10% of the filtered Na^+ and water. Their main clinical use is in the treatment of acute and chronic glaucoma by reducing intraocular pressure since the production of aqueous humour in the eye involves secretion of HCO_3^- by the ciliary body in a process similar to that in the proximal tubule.

The side effects of CA inhibitors include:

- Metabolic acidosis.
- Renal stones.
- Renal K^+ wasting.
- Nervous system effects—paraesthesia and drowsiness.

CA inhibitors should be avoided in patients with liver disease or advanced chronic renal failure.

Thiazide diuretics

These act on the early part of the distal tubule. Since there is more reabsorption of Na^+ in the loop of Henle the loop diuretics are more potent than thiazide diuretics. Thiazides have a role in reducing peripheral vascular resistance, by an unknown mechanism, and are consequently used in the treatment of essential hypertension. They are also indicated in CCF and nephrogenic diabetes insipidus.

The side effects of thiazide diuretics include:

- Hypokalaemic metabolic alkalosis.
- Impaired glucose tolerance.
- Hyperlipidaemia.
- Hyperuricaemia.
- Hypercalcaemia.
- Hyponatraemia.
- Allergic reactions.

Control of hypertension

Control of hypertension can be achieved with:

- Diuretics (i.e. loop diuretics and thiazide diuretics—see above).
- Angiotensin-converting enzyme (ACE) inhibitors.
- β-blockers.
- Vasodilators (i.e. Ca^{2+} channel blockers).

Angiotensin-converting enzyme (ACE) inhibitors

These block ACE, which hydrolyses angiotensin I to angiotensin II. Angiotensin I is inactive and is converted in the lung to angiotensin II; this in turn is converted to angiotensin III in the adrenal gland. Angiotensin·II is a potent vasoconstrictor and aids sodium reabsorption in the tubule. The stimulus for activation of the renin–angiotensin–aldosterone system is reduced renal arteriolar pressure, sympathetic stimulation, and a reduction in the delivery of sodium to the distal tubule (Fig. 4.5).

Any condition resulting in high circulating levels of renin will result in angiotensin-mediated high vascular resistance contributing to hypertension. ACE inhibitors (e.g. captopril, enalapril) inhibit the enzyme peptidyl dipeptidase, which converts angiotensin I to II and therefore lower BP by decreasing TPR. ACE inhibitors may also decrease BP by inhibiting the local (tissue) renin–angiotensin system. ACE inhibitors have been shown to decrease proteinuria and delay the progress of renal disease in diabetic patients. They are also being increasingly used in the treatment of CCF.

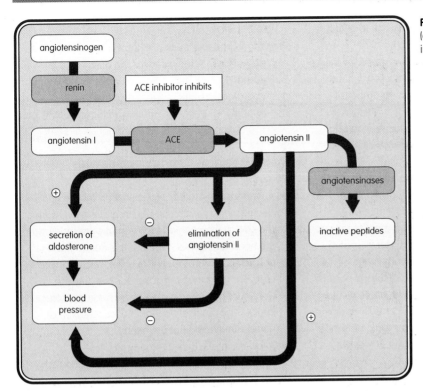

Fig. 4.5 Effects of ACE (angiotensin-converting enzyme) inhibitors.

The side effects of ACE inhibitors include:

- Persistent dry cough.
- Allergic reactions.
- Dose-related proteinuria.
- Taste changes.
- Severe hypotension specially in patients who are hypovolaemic.
- Rashes.
- Acute renal failure in patients with renal artery stenosis.
- Hyperkalaemia.

ACE inhibitors are contraindicated in the final two trimesters of pregnancy because of the risk of:

- Developmental abnormalities in the fetal kidney.
- Oligohydrosaminos.
- Neonatal hypotension and anuria.

Care must be taken in hypertensive patients to ensure thay do not have renal artery stenosis before administering ACE inhibitors; failure to do so could lead to acute renal failure and a lawsuit!

Control of anaemia

Anaemia consists in a fall in the haemoglobin (Hb) concentration to below the reference levels for sex and age. Erythropoietin (EPO) is secreted from the kidneys in response to hypoxia and is the hormone that controls red blood cell production in the bone marrow. In anaemia there is an increase in EPO production in an attempt to increase the number of circulating red blood cells to raise Hb levels. In chronic renal failure there is a relative decrease in the production of endogenous EPO, resulting in a normochromic normocytic anaemia.

The treatment is exogenous (synthetic) EPO, which is produced using recombinant DNA technology. The patients can maintain a haematocrit of 0.35 (normal, 0.45) with subcutaneous or intravenous injection three times a week at a dose of 30–50 U/kg. The aim is to reach an Hb of 10–12 g/dL without the need for blood transfusions.

Side effects of **CAPTOPRIL**
- **Cough.**
- **Allergic reaction.**
- **Proteinuria.**
- **Taste changes.**
- **HypOtension.**
- **Pregnancy—fetal renal failure.**
- **Rash.**
- **Makes you ILL!**

Iron deficiency is the most common cause of failure in EPO treatment and is corrected with oral or intravenous iron supplements. Other reasons for failure include bleeding, malignancy, and infection.

The complications of treatment are thrombotic complications, hypertension, and fitting. These are associated with rapid rises in Hb concentration and haematocrit. Treatment is very expensive.

Management of chronic renal disease

Chronic renal failure (CRF) is associated with many complications. It is usually a progressive disorder leading to end-stage renal failure over months to years. It is important that the underlying disorder is treated aggressively, if possible. There are many other components to the management of CRF. An important part of the management is patient education. All the drug and dietary changes should be carefully explained and where appropriate preparations should be made for dialysis or transplantation (i.e. home or lifestyle adjustments may be required).

Hypertension

Treatment for hypertension is known to reduce the rate of progression in renal disease. The BP is kept below 140/90 mmHg. ACE inhibitors may have an additional nephroprotective effect, especially in diabetic nephropathy. Diuretics are also used to reduce salt and water retention in patients who are not on dialysis.

Dietary restrictions and supplements

These are as follows:

- A decrease in protein intake (low protein diet) to decrease the production of nitrogenous waste; this may delay the onset of symptomatic uraemia and the need for dialysis. Whether this delays the progression remains controversial, but low protein diets are used in some cases for this purpose.
- Control of hyperkalaemia by restriction of potassium intake. Any medication that causes retention of potassium should not be taken.
- A low fat intake is recommended for hyperlipidaemia. Lipid-lowering agents should be considered, although side effects from such drugs are more common in CRF.
- In patients with generalized oedema fluid restriction may be necessary.

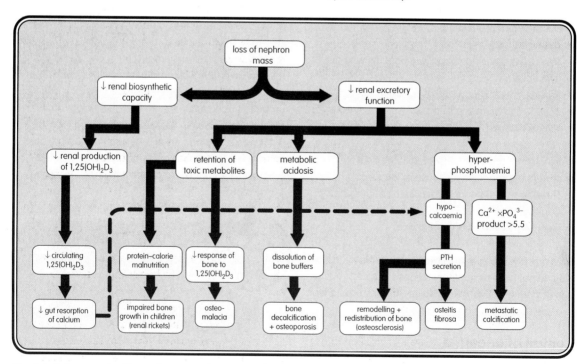

Fig. 4.6 Pathogenesis of bone disease in chronic renal failure.

Management of renal bone disease

The various forms of bone disease in patients with CRF (osteomalacia, secondary and tertiary hyperparathyroidism, osteoporosis, and osteosclerosis) may cause disabling symptoms and it is important that aggressive treatment is given (Fig. 4.6).

The main problems are:

- Decreased glomerular filtration rate (GFR) resulting in increased phosphate, which results in decreased calcium and therefore increased parathyroid hormone (PTH).
- Decreased 1,25-dihdroxycholecalciferol [1,25(OH)$_2$D$_3$] production resulting in decreased calcium.

The aim of treatment is to decrease phosphate levels and increase calcium levels.

Treatment of renal osteodystrophy

Treatment consists of phosphate restriction in the diet and giving phosphate binders to decrease phosphate levels in the body. Calcium carbonate (CaCO$_3$) is a useful phosphate binder since it also increases calcium. Aluminium hydroxide [Al(OH)$_3$] was previously used, but aluminium toxicity has limited its use. Activated vitamin D is used to increase Ca$^+$ and also decreases PTH levels. PTH levels should be checked regularly to ensure that hyperparathyroidism is being controlled. Parathyroidectomy may be required.

Acidosis

Correction of acidosis can be achieved by sodium bicarbonate supplements. The side effects of this treatment include hypertension and oedema. CaCO$_3$ also helps correct acidosis.

Anaemia

See Control of anaemia on p. 71.

Renal replacement therapy

Renal replacement therapy imitates the normal excretory and regulatory functions of the kidney. At best, it provides an equivalent arerage clearance of approximately 10 mL/min (normal GFR, 125 mL/min).

Haemodialysis

This involves the blood being pumped through an artificial kidney called a dialyser. It is passed one side of a semi-permeable membrane, with dialysis fluid being passed in a countercurrent direction on the other side. Dialysis occurs across the semi-permeable membrane removing toxins from the blood. In a typical dialyser:

- Blood flows at 300 mL/min.
- The dialysate flows at 500 mL/min.

Several different synthetic semi-permeable membranes are available with different permeability characteristics. The dialysate is made of purified water and has a solute composition similar to that of plasma, but without any of the waste products, so solutes move along their concentration gradient out of the blood.

Access to the circulation is gained via an arteriovenous fistula, which is surgically constructed. It is usually formed by anastomosing the radial artery and cephalic vein. The venous system 'arterialyses' and the high blood flows required for dialysis can be obtained by 'needling' the venous system. A venous return is used to return blood to the patient. The disadvantages of the arteriovenous fistula include infection and thrombosis.

Dialysis 'dose' can be adjusted by altering the blood flow, the area of the semi-permeable membrane, or the duration of treatment. The average adult with minimal residual renal function requires approximately four hours of treatment three times a week.

Complications of haemodialysis include:

- Hypotension.
- Haemolysis.
- Air embolism.
- Reactions to dialysis membrane.

Haemofiltration

This consists in the removal of plasma water and the solutes dissolved in it, which include sodium, potassium, and urea. This is achieved by convective flow across a high-flux semi-permeable membrane. The fluid is replaced with that of the required biochemical composition. Lactate is the buffer in the replacement fluid. This method is used in acute renal failure (ARF) and chronic renal failure (CRF). It may have the advantage of causing less cardiovascular instability than haemodialysis.

Both haemodialysis and haemofiltration can be used continuously in ARF to ensure slow continuous correction of the fluid and electrolyte balance, especially in patients with haemodynamic instability.

Peritoneal dialysis

This procedure uses the peritoneal membrane as the semi-permeable membrane. This means that there is no need for an arteriovenous fistula for access to the circulation. This requires the insertion of a soft plastic tube through the anterior abdominal wall into the peritoneal cavity. Dialysate is placed into the peritoneum under the influence of gravity. The solutes to be excreted pass into the dialysate along their concentration gradient. Removal of water is achieved by osmosis. Dialysis solutions with high osmolarity will remove more water. Dextrose is commonly employed as an osmotic agent, but will be absorbed by the patient over time. Newer non-absorbable osmotic agents are now available (e.g. glucose polymer). The fluid is regularly exchanged (typically 2 L about 4–5 times a day) to maintain the efficiency of the process. This is called continuous ambulatory peritoneal dialysis (CAPD). CAPD is used in the maintenance dialysis of end-stage renal failure, but technique survival may only be 50% after 5 years due to loss of peritoneal membrane function.

Complications of peritoneal dialysis include:
- Peritonitis (50% is caused by *Staphylococcus epidermidis*).
- Infections around the site of the catheter.

Treatment is with intraperitoneal or intravenous antibiotics.

Other complications include constipation, pleural effusions, and a rare but very serious condition called sclerosing peritonitis.

Contraindications to CAPD are:
- Peritoneal adhesions as a result of peritonitis.
- Abdominal hernia.
- Colostomy.

Renal transplantation

This is the ideal treatment for end-stage renal failure. It restores near-normal renal function and improves quality of life. A donated kidney is anastomosed onto the iliac blood vessels of the recipient and the ureters are inserted into the bladder. The kidney comes from a cadaver or a close living relative. The success of any transplant depends upon:
- ABO group.
- Matching the donor and the recipient for human leucocyte antigen (HLA) types.
- Preoperative blood transfusion.
- Immunosuppressive treatment.

Short-term complications include:
- Acute rejection.
- Operative failure.

Long-term complications include:
- Infection.
- Recurrence of original disease.
- Malignancy, epecially lymphomas.

- For osmotic, potassium sparing, loop, and thiazide diuretics and carbonic anhydrase inhibitors discuss the site of action, mechanism of action, uses, and side effects.
- Outline the use of ACE inhibitors in the treatment of hypertension, indicating their mechanisms of action and side effects.
- Discuss the principles of management of CRF including the management of hypertension, bone disease, acidosis, and anaemia. What is the role of dietary manipulation?
- What are the options in renal replacement therapy and the disadvantages of each?

ORGANIZATION OF THE LOWER URINARY TRACT

Overview

Urine formed in the kidneys collects in the renal pelvis and then passes down the ureters to the bladder and leaves the body through the urethra. The bladder stores the urine, which is intermittently ejected from the body under voluntary control.

Ureters

Anatomy

Fig. 5.1 shows the course of the ureters through the pelvis in a man. The ureters begin as funnel-shaped tubes at the renal pelvis and run over the posterior abdominal wall in front of the external iliac artery down to the pelvic brim (similar course in the female). Each one is 25–30 cm long. Dilatation of the renal pelvis stimulates action potentials in the pacemaker cells of the renal pelvis resulting in peristalsis (Fig. 5.2) Urine is conveyed along the ureters by peristaltic contractions. The ureters are divided up into four regions: renal pelvis, abdominal, pelvic, and intramural regions (Fig. 5.3).

The blood supply to the ureter derives from various sources (i.e. renal, lumbar segmental, gonadal, common iliac, internal iliac, and superior vesical arteries).

Innervation is provided by both sympathetic and parasympathetic nerves. Sensory nerves are from T11–L2 and S2–4, but the motor supply to the muscular wall is unclear. As shown in Fig. 5.3 there are constrictions in the ureters. Stones can get stuck at these constrictions and produce acute pain, which is referred to the skin of T11–L2. Therefore, pain starts in the loin and radiates to the scrotum and penis or to the labium majus.

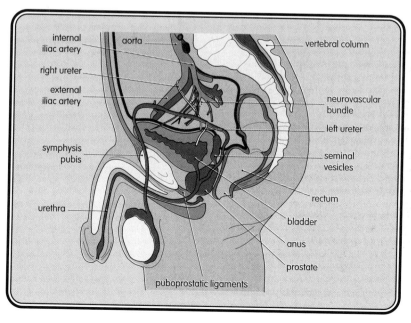

Fig. 5.1 Course of the ureters through the pelvis in a man.

internal iliac artery
aorta
vertebral column
right ureter
external iliac artery
neurovascular bundle
left ureter
symphysis pubis
seminal vesicles
rectum
urethra
bladder
anus
prostate
puboprostatic ligaments

Lymphatic drainage is to the para-aortic lymph nodes.

Histology

The muscular layers are made of smooth muscle (Fig. 5.3) arranged in layers:

- A longitudinal layer just outside the lumen.
- A middle circular layer.
- Another longitudinal layer.

The lumen is lined by urinary epithelium or urothelium, which is folded in the relaxed state allowing the ureter to dilate during the passage of urine.

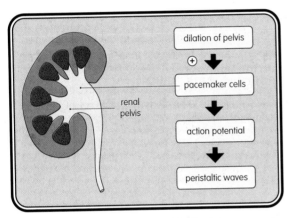

Fig. 5.2 Mechanism of ureteric peristalsis.

Urothelium

The plasma membranes of urothelium are thicker than other cell membranes, stopping interstitial fluid from entering the concentrated urine. Urothelium is impermeable to urine. The cells have highly interdigitating cell junctions, allowing great distension of the epithelium without damaging the surfaces of the cells.

Urinary bladder

Anatomy

The ureters enter the base of the bladder (the upper border of the trigone), which is a highly distensible organ. When empty, it lies in the pelvis and rests on the symphysis pubis and floor of the pelvis. When filled, it enlarges into the abdominal cavity. Partially covered by peritoneum, it has smooth muscular walls and is lined by transitional epithelium or urothelium. The neck of the bladder is relatively immobile and fixed by the puboprostatic and lateral vesical ligament. Fig. 5.4 shows the posterior view of the male bladder, while Fig. 5.5 shows the urinary bladder in the female.

Interior of the bladder

The wall is yellow with rugae (folds) enabling greater expansion with little increase in internal pressure. The base is the trigone, which is a triangular reddish region (Fig. 5.4). This is less mobile and does not wrinkle as the bladder contracts. It is more sensitive to painful stimuli.

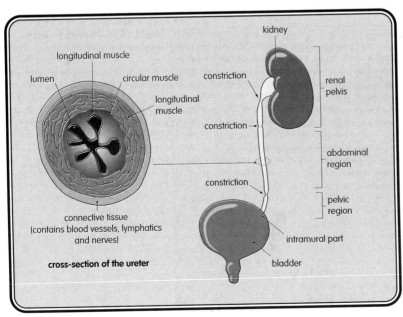

Fig. 5.3 Regions of the ureter and cross-sectional view, highlighting the normal points of reduced diameter at which stones commonly lodge.

The bladder is lined by smooth muscle, which like the ureter is arranged in spiral, long, and circular bundles. It is known as the detrusor muscle. Muscle bundles surround either side of the urethra to form the internal urethral sphincter. Slightly further along the urethra, there is a skeletal muscle sphincter—the external urethral sphincter.

The blood supply to the bladder is provided by the superior and inferior vesical branches of the internal iliac artery. It is drained by the vesical plexus, and by the prostatic venous plexus in the male, which then drain into the internal iliac vein.

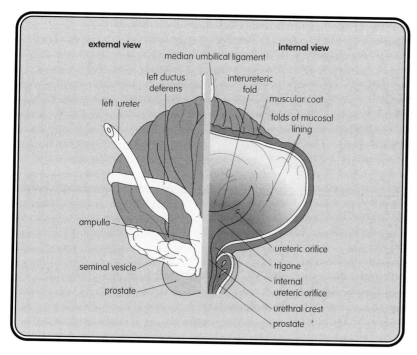

Fig. 5.4 Posterior and interior view of the male bladder.

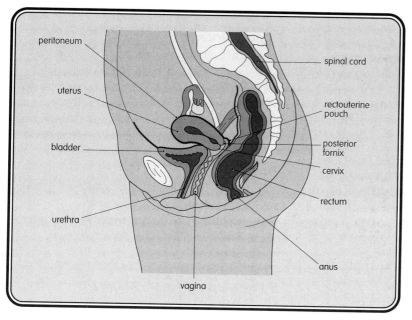

Fig. 5.5 Diagram showing female urinary bladder in the pelvis.

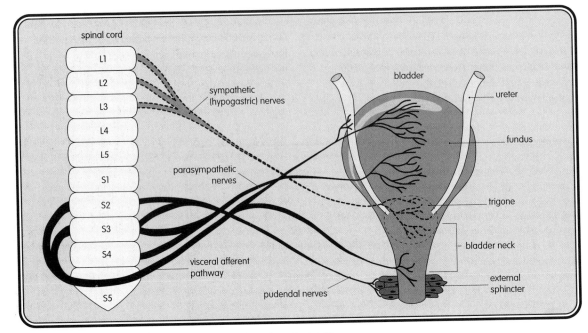

Fig. 5.6 Innervation of the bladder. (From Renal Physiology, 2nd edition. BM Koeppen, B Stanton. Mosby Year Book, 1996.)

Bladder innervation (Fig. 5.6) is both:

- Sensory—gives sensation (awareness) of a full bladder and also pain from disease. If the bladder is empty, the impulses are suppressed.
- Motor—parasympathetic activity results in detrusor muscle stimulation, but inhibits the urethral sphincter allowing micturition. Sympathetic activity inhibits the detrusor muscle and stimulates the urethral sphincter, inhibiting urination.

Lymphatic drainage is to the external iliac nodes.

Histology

This is similar to that of the lower third of the ureter.

Male urethra

The male urethra (Fig. 5.7) is longer than the female urethra (male—20 cm, female—4 cm). Its course is through the neck of bladder, the prostate, floor of pelvis, and perineal membrane to the penis and external urethral orifice at the tip of the glans penis. It has three parts:

- Prostatic urethra.
- Membranous urethra.
- Spongy urethra.

It is innervated by the prostatic plexus and lymphatic drainage is to the internal iliac and deep inguinal nodes.

Histology

The prostatic urethra is lined by urothelium. The rest is lined by stratified or pseudostratified columnar epithelium. The external opening is lined by stratified squamous epithelium.

Female urethra

This is 4 cm long. Its course starts at the neck of the bladder and it passes through the floor of the pelvis and perineal membrane to open into the vestibule just anterior to the opening of the vagina. It is firmly attached to the anterior wall of the vagina. Lymphatics drain to the internal and external iliac lymph nodes.

Prostate

This is a gland lying inferior to the bladder in the male which surrounds the urethra. It measures $4 \times 3 \times 2$ cm and is conical in shape. It is connected to the bladder by connective tissue stroma and has three parts:

- Left lateral lobe.
- Right lateral lobe.
- Middle lobe (see Figs 5.1, 5.4, and 5.7).

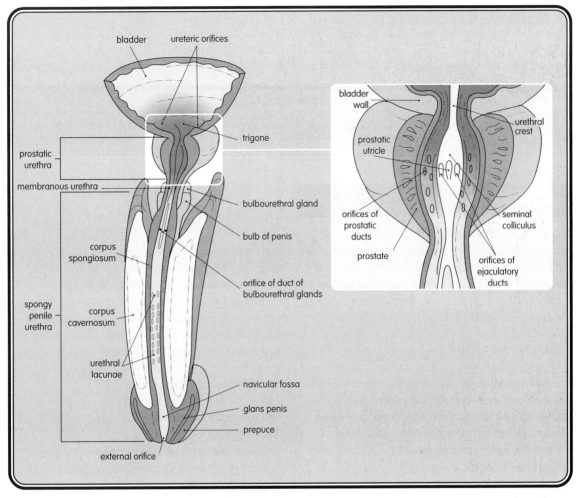

Fig. 5.7 Male urethra.

The prostate has a connective tissue capsule, which is surrounded by a thick sheath from the pelvic fascia. It is influenced by sex hormones resulting in growth during puberty. From the 4th decade onwards, it hypertrophies and nodules of hyperplastic glandular and connective tissue form. As the prostate surrounds the urethra, this can cause obstruction to the flow of urine.

Blood supply to the prostate is via the inferior vesical artery and blood drains to the prostatic plexus, and then to the vesical plexus and internal iliac vein. Innervation is provided by the prostatic plexus. Lymphatics drain to the internal iliac and sacral nodes.

Histology

The prostate consists of glandular lobules. Prostatic glandular epithelium varies from inactive low cuboidal cells to active pseudostratified columnar cells depending upon the degree of androgen stimulation from the testes. Ducts open into the prostatic urethra and secrete 75% of seminal fluid, which is thin, milky, and rich in citric acid and hydrolytic enzymes (e.g. fibrinolysin). This prostatic secretion liquefies coagulated semen after deposition in the female genital tract. The prostate is covered by a stroma and capsule made of dense fibro-elastic connective tissue with many smooth muscle fibres.

MICTURITION

Normal micturition

Micturition is the intermittent voiding of urine stored in the bladder. The inside of the bladder wall is folded so that it can expand and accommodate fluid with little increase in pressure. However, it can only accommodate a certain volume of fluid before an increase in intravesical pressure occurs causing an urge to micturate. Fig. 5.8 shows a normal cystometrogram in which pressure rise is compared to rise in volume in the bladder.

Innervation of the bladder is quite complex (see Fig. 5.6). In infants, micturition is a local spinal reflex where voiding of urine occurs when a critical pressure in the bladder is reached. However, in adults this reflex can be inhibited or facilitated by higher centres in the brain. During micturition:

- Perineal muscles and the external urethral sphincter relax.
- The detrusor muscle contracts.
- Urine is voided.

Bladder distension with urine stimulates bladder stretch receptors, which in turn stimulate the afferent limb of voiding reflex and parasympathetic fibres of the bladder, resulting in the desire to urinate. Higher centre stimulation of the pudendal nerves keeps the external sphincter closed until it is appropraite to urinate. Fig. 5.9 illustrates the voluntary control of micturition. As voiding is voluntary it can be initiated when the bladder is nearly empty and without straining.

Abnormal micturition
Neurological lesions

Urinary continence is affected by various neurological lesions. Fig. 5.10 illustrates various potential points of damage along the micturition pathway.

Lesion in the superior frontal gyrus
This results in:
- Decreased desire to urinate.
- Difficulty stopping micturition once started.

Lesion of afferent nerves from the bladder
A lesion of afferent nerves from the bladder (e.g. due to disease of the dorsal roots such as tabes dorsalis) results

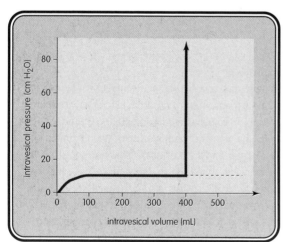

Fig. 5.8 Normal cystometrogram showing the rise in pressure associated with increasing bladder volume.

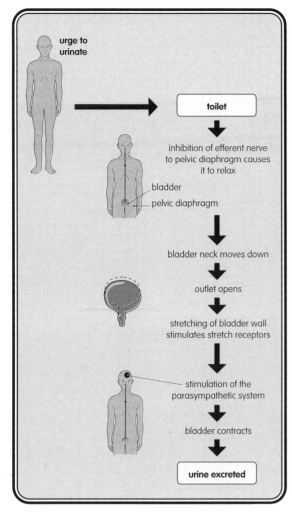

Fig. 5.9 Voluntary control of micturition.

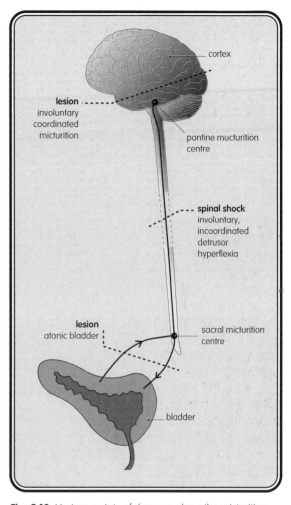

Fig. 5.10 Various points of damage along the micturition pathway.

in no reflex contractions of the bladder and the bladder becomes distended, thin walled, and hypotonic.

Lesion of both afferent and efferent nerves
A lesion of both afferent and efferent nerves (e.g. due to tumour of the cauda equina or filum terminale) results in:
- Initial bladder flaccidity and distension.
- Later increased bladder activity with many contractions and dribbling of urine from the urethra.
- A shrunken bladder with a hypertrophied bladder wall.

Spinal cord lesion
A lesion to the spinal cord (e.g. spinal shock) results in:
- Bladder flaccidity and unresponsiveness with overfill and dribbling of urine (overflow incontinence).

- After shock has passed, the voiding reflex returns, but with no control from higher centres and therefore no voluntary control.
- Occasionally, hyperactive voiding.
- Eventually decreased bladder capacity and wall hypertrophy—spastic neurogenic bladder.

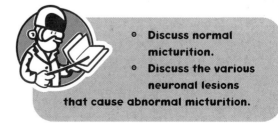

○ **Discuss normal micturition.**
○ **Discuss the various neuronal lesions that cause abnormal micturition.**

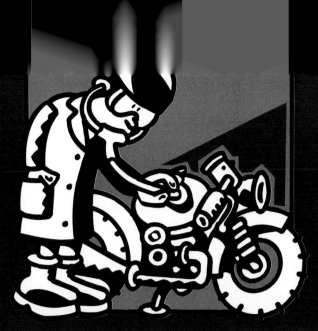

CLINICAL ASSESSMENT

THE HISTORY

Overview

An accurate history is vital as it is the first and most important step in making the correct diagnosis.

- Introduce yourself—shake hands and tell the patient your name and status (i.e. medical student).
- Explain what you are going to do.
- Make sure the patient is comfortable, is at the same level as you, and that there are no barriers between the two of you.
- Put the patient at ease.
- Make sure you listen to the patient and do not look around at for example the room or at your fingers when the patient is talking.
- Make patients feel that they can trust you, so that they can talk to you and tell you their problems—some of which can be very personal.
- Stand back and look around the bedside for clues such as: inhalers, oxygen, dialysis equipment, BM sticks, walking sticks and frames (gives an indication of mobility), sputum pot, cards from the family (show support), and reading material.
- Observe the patient while taking the history for agitation or distress.
- Notice any tremors, difficulties in breathing, speech problems, deafness.

Structure of the history

The following is a simple structure of how the history can be taken. Take details of:

- Name.
- Date of birth.
- Occupation.

Presenting complaint

Get the patient to explain in his or her own words what the trouble seems to be—record the symptoms that are felt by the patient rather than the diagnosis.

History of the presenting complaint

Features of the presenting complaint to ask about are as follows:

- What is the nature of the complaint? Find out about the symptom—for example for pain ask about site, radiation, severity, timing, character (stabbing, burning, pricking), aggravating or relieving factors, and associated symptoms.
- What is the onset and time course of the complaint? Did the symptom occur gradually or suddenly? When did it begin? Is there a pattern and if so, what? Find out whether the symptom is intermittent or constant, how frequently it occurs, how long it lasts for, and its intensity.
- Are there any precipitating or relieving factors? Does anything bring it on or make it worse or better (e.g. position, food, painkillers)? In renal colic, the patient will not be comfortable in any position.
- Are there other relevant or associated symptoms? For example if someone has loin pain, ask about urinary frequency, haematuria, nausea or vomiting, constipation or diarrhoea.
- Has the patient had any previous treatment or investigations for this complaint? Has the patient had a similar problem before and what was done about it?

Particular symptoms relevant to the urinary system are:

- Haematuria (cancer of the renal tract, urinary tract infection, glomerulonephritis).
- Increased frequency (urinary tract infection).
- Poor stream (bladder outflow obstruction—prostatic hypertrophy).
- Nocturia (chronic renal failure or bladder outflow obstruction).

Past medical history

Find out about any illnesses, operations, investigations, and treatments with dates. Get details of past or present medical conditions, such as tuberculosis, asthma, heart conditions, previous strokes, jaundice, epilepsy. Ask about medical conditions associated with renal disease (e.g. diabetes mellitus, hypertension, chronic inflammatory disease, urinary tract infections, rheumatic fever, tonsillitis, previous renal disease).

Drug history

Find out about:

- Any medications being taken, both prescribed and over-the-counter drugs.
- Any known allergies (e.g. penicillin).
- Exposure to toxins (e.g. industrial toxins, lead, hydrocarbons).

Family history

Find out about any illnesses in first-degree relatives, especially renal disease, hypertension, diabetes. Draw a concise diagram of the family tree.

Social history

Find out about:

- Marital status—children and spouse's health.
- Occupation—current job or past job, effect of illness on job, financial problems.
- Accommodation—where does the patient live and who with? Are there any relatives or friends visiting? Can the patient cope at home (i.e. cooking, washing, home surroundings)?
- Diet and exercise.
- Travel—has the patient been abroad recently?
- Alcohol—how many units does the patient drink? (the best way to assess this is to go through the weekly consumption with the patient).
- Smoking—how much? When did the patient start?
- Drugs—'recreational' drugs—how much? How often? For how long?
- Sexual practices.

Review of systems

This is a brief overview of all the body systems (Fig. 6.1).

Summary

Always give a short summary at the end giving:

- The name and age of the patient.
- The presenting complaint and its duration.
- Any important associated symptoms.

Brief overview of the body systems	
General/ body system	**Examination**
general questions	weight loss (carcinoma) appetite night sweats fevers (infections) lumps (carcinoma) fatigue (carcinoma)
cardiorespiratory	chest pain (heart disease) dyspnoea palpitations (heart disease) paroxysmal nocturnal dyspnoea ankle oedema (Na+ and water retention) cough and sputum haemoptysis wheeze (asthma)
gastrointestinal	abdominal pain nausea and vomiting (uraemia) bowel frequency tenesmus or urgency malaena (carcinoma) haematemesis flatulence dysphagia
genitourinary	incontinence* dysuria* haematuria* nocturia* frequency* polyuria* hesitancy* dribbling* menstrual history (cycle and duration, regularity, first day of last menstrual period, number of pregnancies, menarche and menopause)
neurological	fits, blackouts* headaches* sphincter disturbances* dizziness*
musculoskeletal and skin	pain swelling of joints gout rashes/skin conditions*

Fig. 6.1 Brief overview of body systems. *Asterisks indicate those examinations especially relevant to the renal and urinary systems.

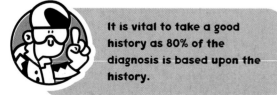

It is vital to take a good history as 80% of the diagnosis is based upon the history.

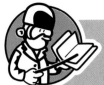

You must be able to take a detailed and accurate history from the patient and maintain the patient's trust in you. Make a list of the things you need to know about:
- **Personal details.**
- **Presenting complaints and history of presenting complaints.**
- **Past medical and drug history.**
- **Family and social history.**

COMMON PRESENTATIONS OF URINARY DISEASE

Introduction

There are numerous presenting complaints in renal disease. In this chapter each will be dealt with individually. Many of these, however, are non-specific and renal disease may be asymptomatic until a very late stage. Therefore it is essential to have a routine screening procedure of:
- Blood pressure measurement.
- Urinalysis.

Haematuria

Blood in the urine may be:
- Microscopic— blood seen only under a microscope or on dipstick analysis.
- Macroscopic— blood seen with the naked eye (over five red blood cells per high-power field).

Causes

Causes of haematuria are listed below (asterisks indicate most common causes).
- Renal causes—glomerular disease such as primary glomerulonephritis (e.g. IgA nephropathy), disorders secondary to systemic illness (e.g. vasculitis, systemic lupus erythematosus—SLE), carcinoma (both renal and transitional cell), trauma, cystic disease, emboli.
- Extrarenal causes—urinary tract infection (UTI)*, ureteral calculi*, prostatic hypertrophy*, carcinoma of the bladder*, renal stone*, trauma, urethritis, catheterization, post-cyclophosphamide.
- Systemic causes—coagulation disorders, sickle-cell trait or disease.
- Others—anticoagulant drugs`.

Dipsticks detect haemoglobin (not red blood cells *per se*) and will give positive results if there is intravascular haemolysis because haemoglobin is freely filtered by glomeruli (haemoglobinuria). This may occur following heavy exercise or with prosthetic heart valves. If haemolysis is severe (i.e. in haemolytic crisis), the urine may become red.

Other conditions may cause a red–brown discoloration of the urine that may be confused with haematuria [e.g. porphyria, myoglobinuria, ingestion of some foods (beetroot) or drugs (phenolphthalein)].

Diagnostic approach

Fig. 6.2 shows the common sites of lesions causing haematuria and a diagnostic approach to the causes of haematuria is shown in Fig. 6.3. An algorithm for the investigation of heamaturia when the IVP or ultrasound result is abnormal is given in Fig. 6.4. Additional points are shown in Fig. 6.5.

Uraemia

Uraemia is the accumulation of nitrogenous metabolic waste products in the blood (i.e. urea and creatinine). The kidneys are unable to filter and excrete these products. If this disorder develops rapidly within a few days, it is known as acute renal failure (ARF). If it occurs over a period of months to years, it is known as chronic renal failure (CRF).

Causes

Causes of uraemia can be classified as prerenal, renal, and postrenal.

Prerenal causes of ARF are:
- Hypovolemia (e.g. shock, burns, dehydration, sepsis, haemorrhage), resulting in decreased effective circulating volume.
- Reduced effective circulating volume (e.g. in congestive cardiac failure, liver disease).

87

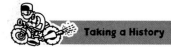

- Drugs altering renal haemodynamics (e.g. non-steroidal anti-inflammatory drugs—NSAIDs, angiotensin-converting enzyme inhibitors, antihypertensives, cyclosporin).
- Renal artery stenosis or emboli.

Renal causes of ARF are:

- Acute tubular necrosis—any prerenal cause left untreated; drug toxicity (e.g. gentamycin, acyclovir, methotrexate); and toxins (e.g. myoglobinuria and lipopolysaccharide in Gram-negative sepsis).
- Acute glomerulonephritis.
- Acute interstitial nephritis (due to drugs, infections, hypercalcaemia, multiple myeloma).
- Vasculitis.
- Hypertension.
- Emboli (such as thrombi, cholesterol).
- Acute cortical necrosis (severe shock left untreated).

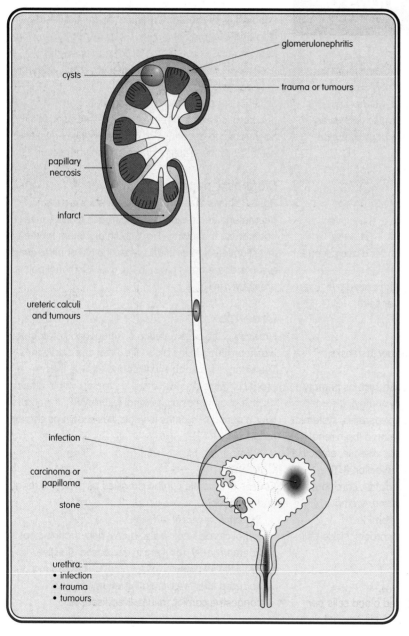

Fig. 6.2 Common sites of lesions causing haematuria.

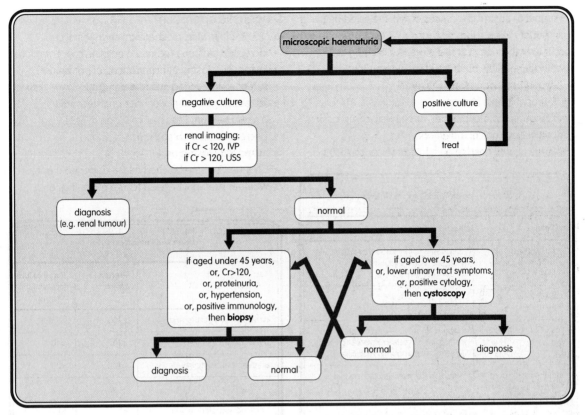

Fig. 6.3 Investigation of haematuria. (Cr, creatinine; IVP, intravenous pyelography; USS, ultrasonography.)

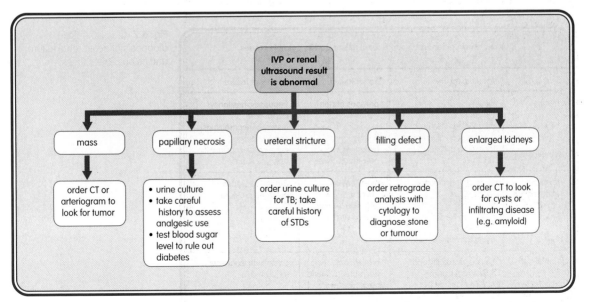

Fig. 6.4 Investigation of haematuria when the IVP or ultrasound result is abnormal. (CT, computerized tomography; IVP, intravenous pylography; STDs, sexually transmitted diseases; TB, tuberculosis) (From Clinical Medicine, 2e by HL Green, Mosby Year Book, 1996.)

89

Postrenal or obstructive causes of ARF are listed below. It is important to note that, to cause ARF, obstruction must occur to both kidneys or to a single functioning kidney.

- Bladder outflow obstruction (benign prostatic hypertrophy or urethral strictures).
- Retroperitoneal fibrosis.
- Tumour (prostate, bladder, or extrinsic compression by gynaecological malignancy).
- Stone (would need to be bilateral to cause ARF).

Diagnostic approach

In ARF, the following biochemical changes occur:
- Increased plasma urea and creatinine concentrations.
- Increased plasma concentrations of potassium.
- Acidosis and an increased anion gap.
- Increased plasma phosphate and decreased plasma calcium (less marked than in CRF).
- Decreased plasma sodium.
- Increased plasma urate.
- Changes in urine biochemistry—dependent upon whether prerenal or renal failure exists (Fig. 6.6).

Urine analysis—possible findings and interpretation	
Findings	**Possible diagnoses**
clots in urine	carcinoma of the bladder or kidney; clot colic is also a feature of IgA nephropathy
albuminuria and haematuria	intrinsic renal disease
red blood cell casts	glomerulonephritis—red cell casts are pathognomic of active glomerular bleeding (e.g. IgA, nephropathy, vasculitis)
haematuria, pyuria and white blood cell casts	renal tubulointerstitial disease; this is a non-specific diagnosis (i.e. pyelonephritis)
dysmorphic red cells	glomerular bleeding (i.e. glomerulonephritis)

Fig. 6.5 Urine analysis—findings and their interpretations.

Urine biochemistry results		
Test	**Prerenal failure**	**Renal failure (acute tubular necrosis)**
urine osmolality (mOsm/kg H_2O)	>500	<350
urine sodium (mmol/L)	<20	>40
urine/serum creatinine	>40	<20
urine/serum osmolality	>1.5	<1.2
fractional excreted sodium	<1	>1
renal failure index	↑urea >creatinine	↑urea ↑creatinine

Fig. 6.6 Urine biochemistry results.

Fig. 6.7 Clues to help in diagnosis of acute renal failure and its possible causes.

Clues to help in diagnosis of acute renal failure and its possible causes			
	Prerenal failure	**Renal failure**	**Postrenal failure**
History	thirst; weight loss; potential for volume loss (e.g. surgery, diuretics) ineffective circulating volume	previous abnormal urinalysis; exposure to toxic agents; hypertension; new medications	frequency; hesitancy; nocturia; history of nephrolithiasis or neoplasms; renal colic especially if only one kidney
Physical examination	signs of dehydration; hypotension; hypovolaemia; ↓ BP = postural drop; ↑ pulse; ↓ jugular venous pulse	hypertension; physical signs (e.g. skin lesions of vasculitis)	distended bladder; enlarged prostate
Urinalysis	↑ urine osmolality and high specific gravity; ↓ urine Na+ and fractional excreted Na+; ↑ urine:serum creatinine	proteinuria; haematuria; pyuria; renal tubular epithelial cells in urinary sediment; casts and their nature	crystalluria (suggests renal calculus)

In addition, some serological tests may help to indicate a diagnosis:
- Antinuclear antibodies (ANA)—lupus nephritis.
- Cryoglobulin titre—cryoglobulinaemia.
- Complement levels—lupus nephritis, membranoproliferative and acute glomerulonephritis.

Fig. 6.7 gives clues to help in the diagnosis of ARF and its possible causes.

Proteinuria

Proteinuria is the presence of excess protein in the urine. It is usually assessed using a dipstick, which should be negative for protein in normal individuals. Proteinuria can be expressed as the protein concentration on a spot urine or the amount excreted per day (assessed using a 24-hour urine collection). Urine usually contains <20mg/L of albumin and 24-hour urinary protein excretion is <200mg (exact values may vary from laboratory to laboratory according to methods used to measure protein). Microalbuminuria is a term used to describe the presence of excess urinary protein, but in amounts insufficient to cause a positive dipstick analysis (sensitivity of most dipsticks is 300mg/L). The presence of protein predicts nephropathy in diabetes and increased cardiovascular risk in hypertension and ischaemic heart disease.

Causes

Causes of proteinuria are:
- Diabetic nephropathy.
- Glomerulonephritis.
- Urinary tract infection.
- Hypertension.
- Myeloma.
- Amyloid.
- Pregnancy.
- Postural proteinuria.
- Exercise.
- Congestive cardiac failure.
- Pyrexia.
- Vaginal mucus contaminant.

Nephrotic syndrome

This is characterized by heavy proteinuria (usually >3 g/day) sufficient to cause a decrease in serum albumin and hence oedema. There is also an increase in cholesterol. Primary nephrotic syndrome results from diseases arising in the glomerulus. It can be due to:
- Commonly, minimal change glomerulonephritis,

membranous glomerulonephritis, membranoproliferative glomerulonephritis, focal segmental glomerulosclerosis.
- Rarely, other types of glomerulonephritis.

Causes of secondary nephrotic syndrome are diabetic nephropathy, drugs (captopril, NSAIDs), amyloidosis, and vasculitis (SLE).

Diagnostic approach

The diagnostic approach to proteinuria is shown in Fig. 6.8.

Hyperuricaemia

Hyperuricaemia is an excess of uric acid (end-product of purine degradation) in the serum.

Causes

Causes of hyperuricaemia are:
- Overproduction of uric acid due to increased biosynthesis of uric acid, increased turnover of tissue nucleic acids, or increased intake of purine precursors.
- Underexcretion of uric acid due to decreased glomerular filtration rate (GFR), decreased tubular secretion, or increased tubular reabsorption.
- A combination of the two above.

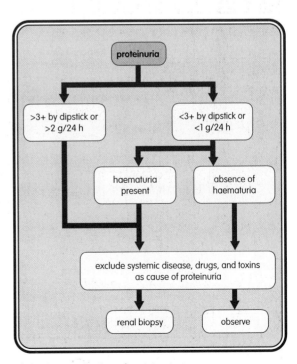

Fig. 6.8 Investigation of proteinuria.

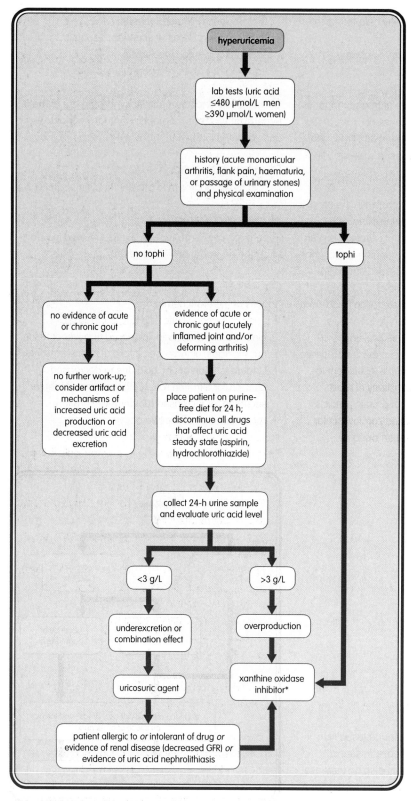

Fig. 6.9 Investigation of hyperuricaemia. *In tophaceous gout, both a xanthine oxidase inhibitor and a uricosuric agent may be needed; xanthine oxidase is an enzyme in the metabolic pathway that produces urate from purines. (From Clinical Medicine, 2e by HL Green, Mosby Year Book, 1996.)

Diagnostic approach

An algorithm for the investigation of hyperuricaemia is given in Fig. 6.9.

Kidney stones

Kidney stone disease arises from the formation and movement of stones within the urinary tract. Different types of stones can form:

- Calcium-containing stones (most common) made of calcium oxalate, hydroxyapatite, brushite.
- Uric acid stones.
- Struvite or infection stones.
- Cysteine stones.

Causes

Causes of kidney stones are:

- Hypercalciuria.
- Hyperuricaemia.
- Hyperuricosuria.
- Hypercalcaemia.
- Hyperoxaluria.
- Infection.
- Cystinuria.
- Renal tubular acidosis.
- Renal disease (e.g. polycystic kidneys).
- Dehydration—a concentrated urine forms increasing the tendency for stone formation.

Diagnostic approach

History

Ask about the following:

- Diet—high dietary calcium intake (e.g. milk, cheese); high salt instake (calcium is excreted in parallel with sodium in the kidney); high dietary oxalate intake (e.g. spinach, rhubarb, tea).
- Fluid intake and urine volume.
- Chronic diarrhoea—Crohn's disease or dehydration.
- Personal or family history of gout.
- Family history of renal calculi.
- Bacterial infection of the urinary tract.
- Medications—check for antacid therapy (contains large amounts of absorbable calcium) and long-term antibiotic therapy.
- Past urological history.

Symptoms

Pain is usually localized to one quadrant radiating down to the groin, usually from loin to groin. There is nausea and vomiting.

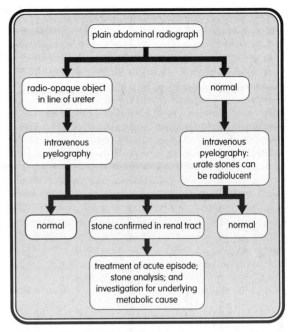

Fig. 6.10 Management of renal calculi.

Examination and investigation

Examinations and investigations for renal calculi (Fig. 6.10) should include:

- Looking for clinical evidence of gout.
- Excluding hypercalcaemia and investigating cause if found (e.g. primary hyperparathyroidism).
- Urinalysis for excess calcium, oxalate, urate, or cysteine.
- Stone analysis (ask patient to retain voided stones).
- Imaging studies, including radiography of the abdomen (showing the kidneys, ureters, and bladder), intravenous urography, and ultrasonography (less helpful, but may show dilatation of obstructed kidney).

Fig. 6.11 shows an algorithm for urinary investigations of a patient with calcium kidney stones.

Treatment

The mainstay of treatment for all stone types is to increase fluid intake. Thiazides are useful in hypercalcuria as they decrease calcium excretion. Allopurinol is used for hyperuricaemia, penicillamine for cysteinuria.

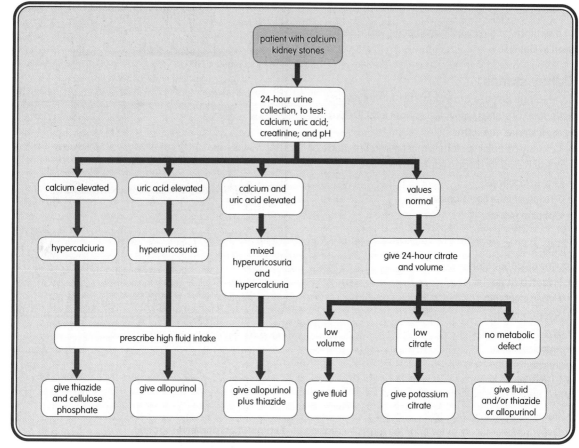

Fig. 6.11 Urinary investigations of a patient with calcium kidney stones. (From Clinical Medicine, 2e by HL Green, Mosby Year Book, 1996.)

Disorders of serum sodium

Hyponatraemia

In hyponatraemia serum sodium concentration is less than 130 mmol/L and there is a decreased ratio of solute to water in the ECF.

Causes

The causes of hyponatraemia are:
- Diuretics (mainly thiazides).
- Water excess.
- Increased antidiuretic hormone (ADH) secretion.
- Water retention.
- Increased plasma osmolarity (e.g. caused by mannitol, glucose).
- Increased protein or lipids (pseudohyponatraemia).

Diagnostic approach

The diagnostic approach to hyponatraemia is shown in Fig. 6.12.

Hypernatraemia

In hypernatraemia the serum sodium is higher than 140 mmol/L and there is an increase in solute to water ratio in body fluids and increased serum osmolality (>300 mOsm/kg).

Causes

The causes of hypernatraemia are:
- Osmotic diuresis (e.g. uncontrolled diabetes).
- Fluid loss without replacement (sweating, burns, vomiting).
- Diabetes insipidus.
- Incorrect intravenous replacement (i.e. hypertonic fluids).
- Primary aldosteronism.

Diagnostic approach

The diagnostic approach to hypernatraemia is shown in Fig. 6.13.

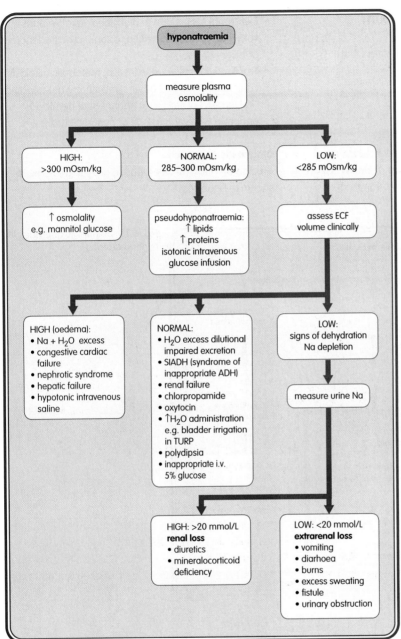

Fig. 6.12 Diagnostic approach to hyponatraemia. (ECF, extracellular fluid; SIADH, syndrome of inappropriate ADH secretion; TURP, transurethral resection of prostate.)

hyponatraemia

measure plasma osmolality

HIGH: >300 mOsm/kg

NORMAL: 285–300 mOsm/kg

LOW: <285 mOsm/kg

↑ osmolality e.g. mannitol glucose

pseudohyponatraemia: ↑ lipids ↑ proteins isotonic intravenous glucose infusion

assess ECF volume clinically

HIGH (oedema):
• Na + H_2O excess
• congestive cardiac failure
• nephrotic syndrome
• hepatic failure
• hypotonic intravenous saline

NORMAL:
• H_2O excess dilutional impaired excretion
• SIADH (syndrome of inappropriate ADH)
• renal failure
• chlorpropamide
• oxytocin
• ↑H_2O administration e.g. bladder irrigation in TURP
• polydipsia
• inappropriate i.v. 5% glucose

LOW: signs of dehydration Na depletion

measure urine Na

HIGH: >20 mmol/L **renal loss**
• diuretics
• mineralocorticoid deficiency

LOW: <20 mmol/L **extrarenal loss**
• vomiting
• diarhoea
• burns
• excess sweating
• fistule
• urinary obstruction

Disorders of serum potassium
Hypokalaemia
In hypokalaemia serum potassium is less than 3.5 mmol/L.

Causes
Hypokalaemia can result from:
- Renal losses due to diuretics, excess mineralocorticoids, magnesium deficiency, renal tubular defects (e.g. renal tubular acidosis), reduced intake, or metabolic alkalosis (e.g. vomiting).
- Extrarenal losses due to diarrhoea, laxative abuse, vomiting, profuse sweating, colonic villous adenoma, or biliary drainage.
- Transcellular shift due to insulin, metabolic alkalosis, catecholamines and other sympathomimetics, rapid proliferation of cells (e.g. treatment of pernicious anaemia with vitamin B_{12}), or periodic paralysis.

Diagnostic approach
An algorithm for the investigation of hypokalaemia is shown in Fig. 6.14.

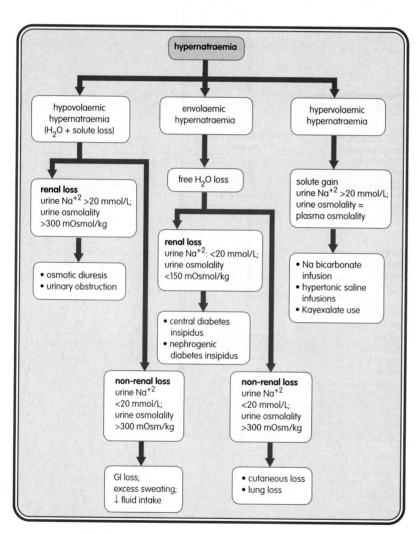

Fig. 6.13 Diagnostic approach to hypernatraemia.

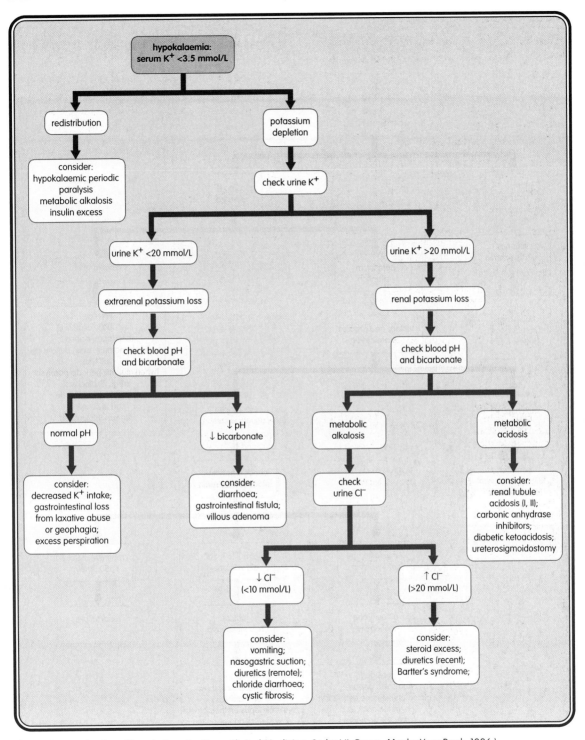

Fig. 6.14 Investigation of hypokalaemia. (From Clinical Medicine, 2e by HL Green, Mosby Year Book, 1996.)

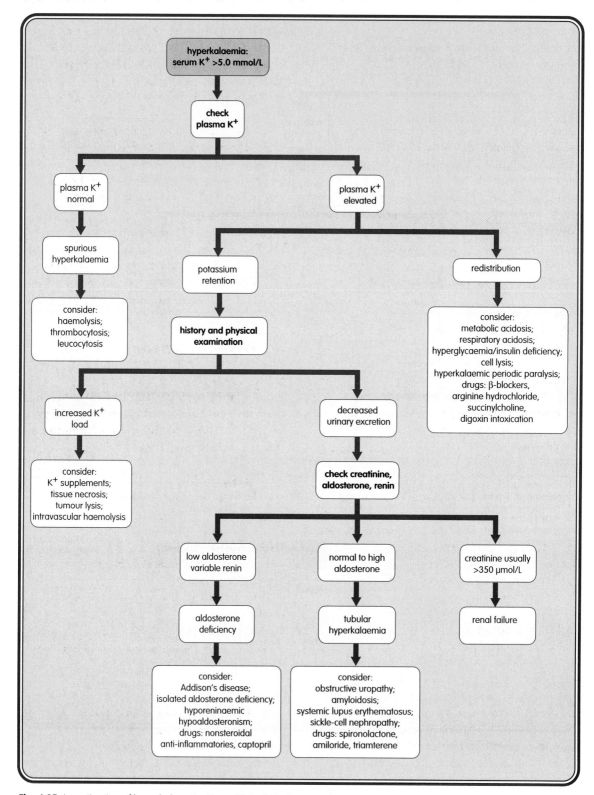

Fig. 6.15 Investigation of hyperkalaemia. (From Clinical Medicine, 2e by HL Green, Mosby Year Book, 1996.)

Hyperkalaemia

In hyperkalaemia serum potassium is higher than 5.5 mmol/L.

Causes

Hyperkalaemia can result from:

- Reduced renal excretion due to renal failure, mineralocorticoid deficiency (e.g. Addison's disease), potassium sparing diuretics, or renal tubular defects.
- Increased load due to diet or tissue breakdown.
- Transcellular shift due to metabolic acidosis, insulin deficiency, exercise, or drugs (e.g. digoxin).
- Pseudohyperkalaemia due to efflux from cells (e.g. trauma during venepuncture, prolonged storage, haemolysis), thrombolysis, or leucocytosis.

Diagnostic approach

An algorithm for the investigation of hyperkalaemia is shown in Fig. 6.15.

Chronic renal failure

Chronic renal failure (CRF) is irreversible impaired renal function. It can result from renal disease or be secondary to other systemic diseases.

Causes

Causes of CRF are:

- Renal—glomerulonephritis, chronic pyelonephritis, obstruction, polycystic kidneys, interstitial nephritis, amyloid, myeloma, renal vascular disease, Alport's syndrome, analgesic nephropathy.
- Extrarenal—diabetes mellitus, hypertension (expecially if accelerated—malignant), SLE, gout, hypercalcaemia.

Diagnostic approach

The diagnostic approach to CRF can involve:

- Urine—urinalysis (haematuria, glycosuria, proteinuria), microscopy (white cells, eosinophilia, granular casts, red cell casts, red cells), biochemistry (24-hour creatinine clearance, 24-hour protein excretion, urinary electrolytes, osmolality, protein electrophoresis).
- Blood—urea and creatinine, electrolytes, glucose, calcium (decreased), phosphate (increased), urate (increased), protein, osmolality, full blood count, erythrocyte sedimentation rate (ESR), protein electrophoresis, auto-antibody screen, complement components, test for sickle-cell disease.
- Radiology—ultrasound, CT, plain radiography of the abdomen. Hand radiographs may show evidence of osteodystrophy.
- Renal biopsy—if kidneys are of normal size and the cause of CRF is not clear from other investigations.

Urethral discharge

A urethral discharge is secretion passed through the urethra at times other than voiding. The secretion may be clear, purulent, or bloody.

Causes

Causes of urethral discharge are:

- Non-infectious—irritation (mechanical or chemical), urethral stricture, non-bacterial prostatitis, phimosis, urethral diverticulum, urethral carbuncle.
- Infectious—gonococcal urethritis, non-gonococcal urethritis (i.e. *Chlamydia trachomatis, Trichomonas vaginalis,* herpes simplex virus).

Diagnostic approach

An algorithm for diagnosing urethral discharge is given in Fig. 6.16.

Dysfunctional voiding

In dysfunctional voiding there are abnormal characteristics of voiding. They can be:

- Irritative, producing frequency, nocturia, urgency, and dysuria.
- Obstructive with symptoms of hesitancy, diminished force, dribbling, and increased residual urine.

Causes

Irritative bladder symptoms can be due to:

- Local abnormality with decreased bladder capacity. This can be due to infection, inflammation, or fibrosis. Causes include acute

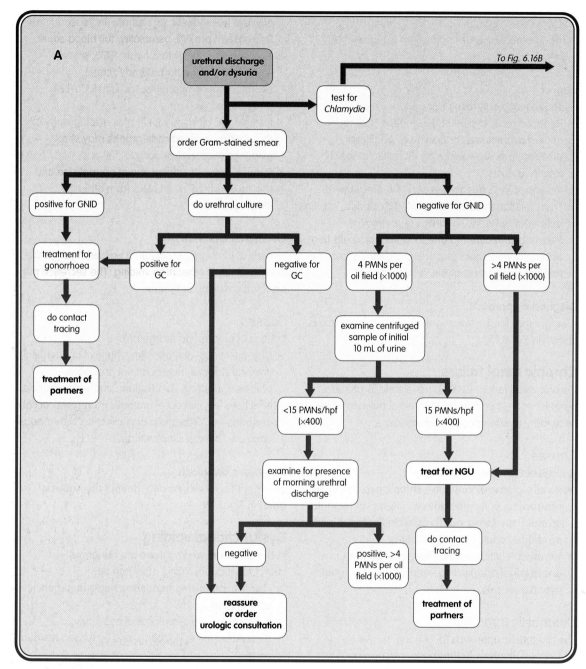

Fig. 6.16A Diagnosing urethral discharge. (GU, gonococcal urethritis; GNID, Gram-negative intracellular diplococci; hpf, high-power field; NGU, non-gonococcal urethritis; PMNs, polymorphonuclear leucocytes.) (From Clinical Medicine, 2e by HL Green, Mosby Year Book, 1996.)

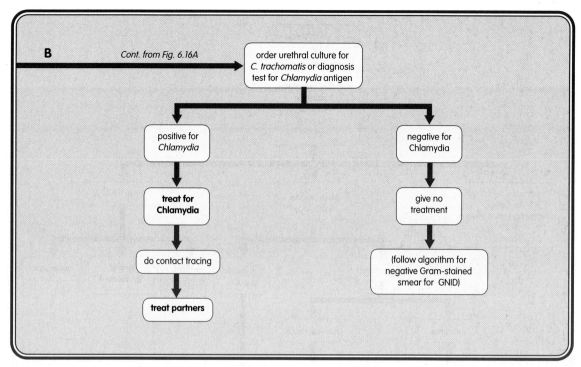

Fig. 6.16B Continued from Fig. 6.16A.

pyogenic infections, chronic infections (i.e. tuberculosis), chlamydia, chronic fungi, foreign body, stone, trauma, radiation, cyclophosphamide, interstitial cystitis, and chronic obstruction.

• Neurological abnormality, such as damage to the cortex or upper spinal cord. Causes include stroke, cerebral atrophy, and multiple sclerosis.

Obstructive bladder symptoms are commoner in men than in women due to the longer urethra, which can be easily compressed or narrowed. Causes are given in Fig. 6.17.

Diagnostic approach
Algorithms for the aetiology of irritative and obstructive bladder symptoms in dysfunctional voiding are given in Figs 6.18 and 6.19.

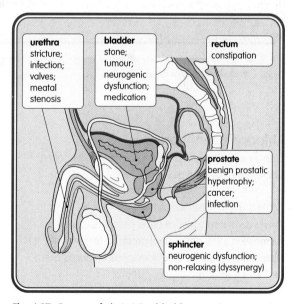

Fig. 6.17 Causes of obstructive bladder symptoms.

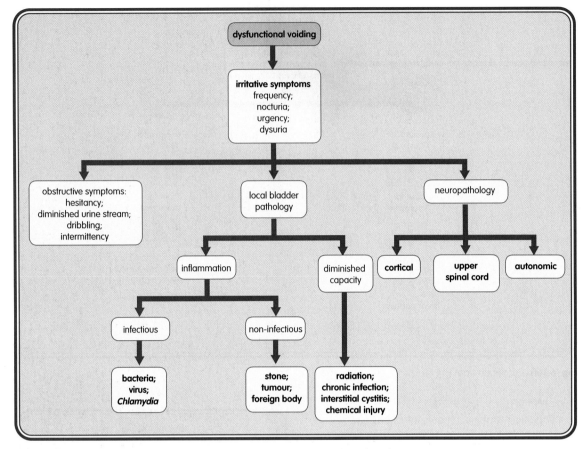

Fig. 6.18 Causes of irritative symptoms in dysfunctional voiding. (From Clinical Medicine, 2e by HL Green, Mosby Year Book, 1996.)

Urinary incontinence

Urinary incontinence is the involuntary loss of urine There are different types.

Stress incontinence

This is involuntary loss of urine associated with an increase in intra-abdominal pressure (e.g. cough). It is also called sphincter insufficiency. The causes are:
- Pelvic floor laxity.
- Inherent weakness of the bladder neck.
- Surgery affecting the urethra or prostate causing damage or weakness to the external sphincter.

Urge incontinence

This is involuntary loss of urine when the urge to void is noticed. There is an urgent 'need to go'. It is also called detrusor instability. The causes are:

- Inflammation or infection of the lower urinary tract.
- Bladder hyperreflexia.
- Stroke.
- Parkinson's disease.
- Alzheimer's disease.
- Brain tumour.
- Old age.
- Herniated disc.
- Detrusor overactivity caused by a foreign body, stone, or urethritis.
- Benign prostatic hypertrophy and obstruction (may cause bladder hypersensitivity).
- Loop diuretics.
- Cough or sneeze.

Overflow incontinence

Overflow incontinence is involuntary loss of urine when

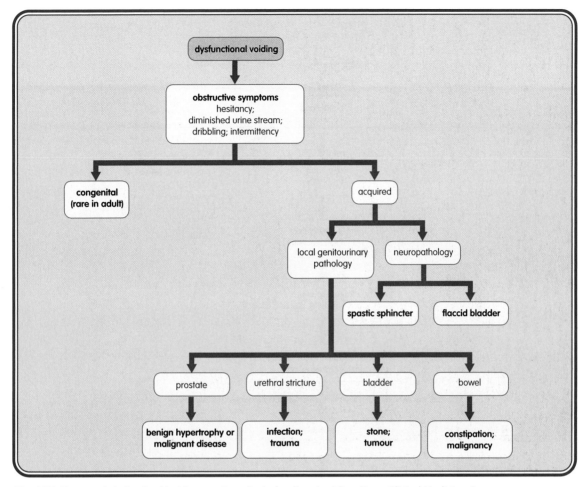

Fig. 6.19 Causes of obstructive bladder symptoms in dysfunctional voiding. (From Clinical Medicine, 2e by HL Green, Mosby Year Book, 1996.)

the bladder is full. It is also called paradoxical incontinence. The causes are:

- Outlet obstruction.
- Underactive detrusor muscle.
- Enlarged prostate.
- Bladder neck stricture.
- Faecal impaction.
- Urethral stricture.
- α-adrenergic agonists.
- Intra- or postoperative overdistension.
- Use of anticholinergics, calcium channel blockers, sedatives.
- Bladder denervation following surgery.

Total incontinence

This is continuous loss of urine with no voluntary control.

The causes are:

- Congenital.
- Secondary to paraplegia, multiple sclerosis, spina bifida.
- Trauma to the external sphincter, bladder neck, and perineal muscles.
- Fistula secondary to radiation, surgery, tumour, invasive neoplasms, obstetric injury.

Reflex incontinence

This is involuntary intermittant loss of urine.

Functional incontinence

This is wetting because severe cognitive impairment or mobility limitations prevent use of the toilet; for example, there may be difficulty in reaching the toilet, difficulty in undressing, or lack of facilities.

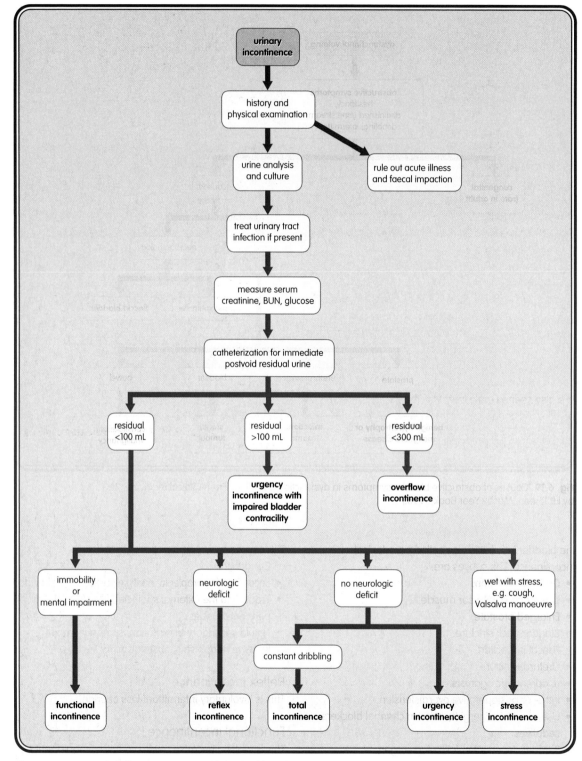

Fig. 6.20 Investigation of urinary incontinence. (BUN, blood urea nitrogen; UTI, urinary tract infection.) ((From Clinical Medicine, 2e by HL Green, Mosby Year Book, 1996.)

Mixed incontinence
In mixed incontinence there is more than one type of problem. This disorder occurs in the elderly.

Nocturnal enuresis—bedwetting
The causes of nocturnal enuresis can be primary (since birth) or secondary (acquired). Both can be due to:
- Uninhibited bladder activity.
- Urinary infection.
- Neurological disease.
- Obstruction.

Diagnostic approach
Fig. 6.20 shows an algorithm for the investigation of urinary incontinence.

Urinary tract infection
Urinary tract infection (UTI) [i.e. $>10^5$ colony-forming units (CFU)/mL] occurs with or without leucocytes. It is most common in adult women because bacteria can readily access the urinary tract through the short female urethra. UTI results from migration of bacteria through the urethra into the bladder, ureter, and kidney. UTIs are also seen in male infants with congenital obstruction and in elderly men with acquired prostatic obstruction. Different sites of the urinary tract may be affected as follows:

- Kidney, resulting in pyelonephritis.
- Bladder, resulting in cystitis.
- Prostate, resulting in prostatitis.
- Urethra, resulting in urethritis.

Risk factors for UTI are:
- Diabetes mellitus.
- Pregnancy.
- Impaired voiding (due to obstruction).
- Genitourinary malformations.
- Sexual intercourse.
- Stones.
- Neurogenic bladder.
- Intact male foreskin.

The main organisms involved are:
- *Escherichia coli.*
- *Staphylococcus saprophyticus.*
- *Proteus* spp.
- *Klebsiella* spp.
- *Enterobacter* spp.
- *Pseudomonas* spp.
- *Enterococcus* spp.

Diagnostic approach
Algorithms for the investigation of UTI are given in Figs. 6.21–6.23.

For the following abnormalities, discuss the differential diagnosis and indicate what investigations should be carried out to obtain an accurate diagnosis:
- Haematuria.
- Proteinuria.
- Uraemia.
- Hyperuricaemia.
- Kidney stones.
- Abnormal serum sodium.
- Abnormal serum potassium.
- Chronic renal failure.
- Urethral discharge.
- Dysfunctional voiding.
- Urinary incontinence.
- Urinary tract infection.

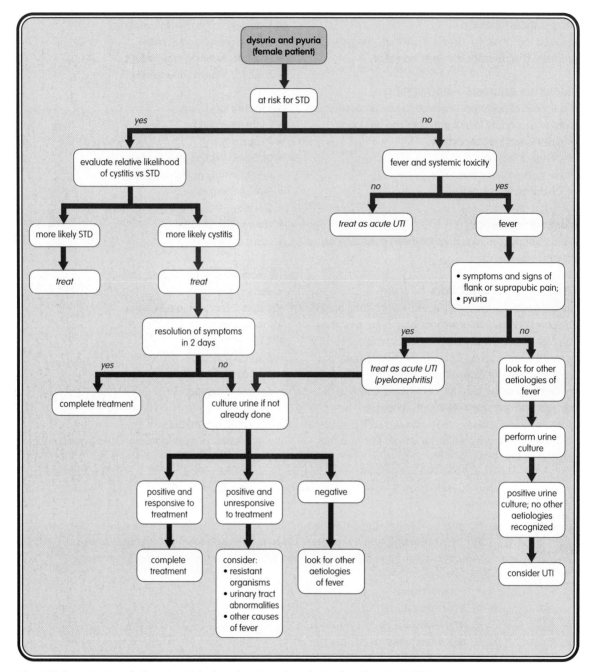

Fig. 6.21 Investigation of urinary tract infection: dysuria and pyuria in a female patient. (STD, sexually transmitted disease; UTI, urinary tract infection.) (From Clinical Medicine, 2e by HL Green, Mosby Year Book, 1996.)

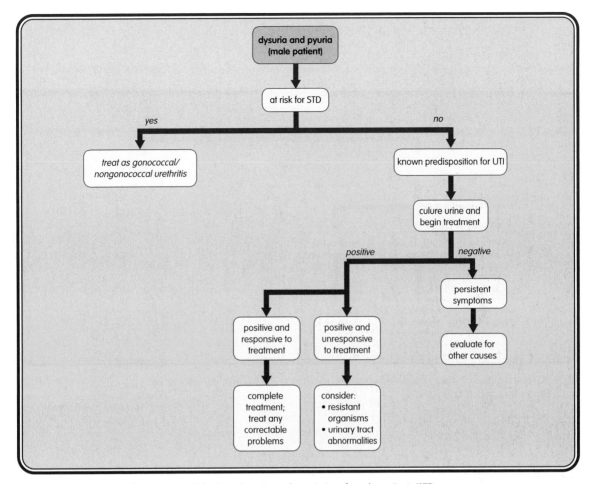

Fig. 6.22 Investigation of urinary tract infection: dysuria and pyuria in a female patient. (STD, sexually transmitted disease; UTI, urinary tract infection.) (From Clinical Medicine, 2e by HL Green, Mosby Year Book, 1996.)

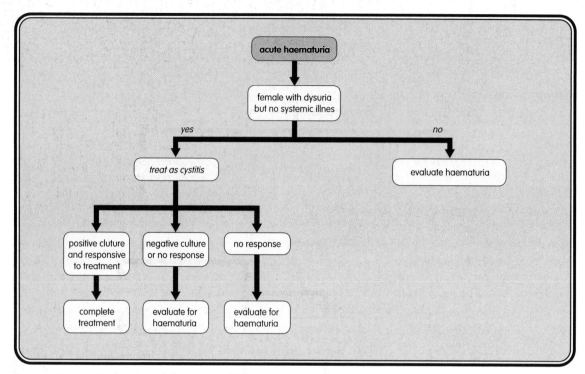

Fig. 6.23 Investigation of urinary tract infection: acute haematuria. (From Clinical Medicine, 2e by HL Green, Mosby Year Book, 1996.)

GENERAL INSPECTION

Overview

Whenever examining someone it is very important to remember the following points:

- Always introduce yourself to the patient.
- Observe the patient carefully before you examine as this will give you a general impression of the patient's condition.
- Look around the patient for any extra clues—urinalysis strips, sputum pot or oxygen mask.
- Position the patient appropriately for the examination—at 45 degrees for cardiovascular or respiratory system examination or lying flat for abdominal examination.
- Expose appropriate part of body and ensure the patient is comfortable.
- Stand back and observe the patient from the end of the bed before you touch the patient.

When taking a history always introduce yourself to the patient, observe the patient carefully, and look around the patient for any clues.

- Look to see if the patient is conscious or looks well, is in pain, appears anxious or depressed, smells of urine, or has any major skeletal abnormalities.
- In renal patients special attention should be made to stature (Fig. 7.1), any obvious skin pigmentation (Fig. 7.2), and fat distribution.

Face & neck and respiratory signs related to renal disease are listed respectively in Figs 7.3 and 7.4, while Fig. 7.5 lists the signs related to dialysis equipment.

Fig. 7.1 Signs related to stature and weight in renal disease. (BMI body mass index; CRF, chronic renal failure.)

Signs related to stature and weight in renal disease		
Test	**Sign**	**Diagnostic inference**
stature	short stature	seen in patients who had CRF in childhood: growth is impaired due to an abnormal response to growth hormone and puberty is delayed
weight and height • measure weight and height • compare with ideal weight for height and calculate body mass index (BMI)	BMI = weight ÷ (height)^2 • underweight if BMI <19 kg/m^2 • obese if BMI >30 kg/m^2 an increase in weight can be due to oedema	• oedema of nephrotic syndrome can be confused with obesity • a low BMI is seen in CRF due to anorexia and malnutrition
oedema (tissue swelling due to accumulation of excess fluid)	• periorbital oedema (swelling of the eyelid) • general puffiness of the face • oedema of the legs • sacral oedema	renal causes of oedema: • acute glomerulonephritis • nephrotic syndrome • renal failure

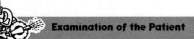

Signs related to skin colour in renal disease		
Test	**Sign**	**Diagnostic inference**
pallor	conjunctivae are pale	in CRF, there is a decrease in erythropoietin causing an anaemia with normal iron concentration; other causes of anaemia are iron, vitamin B_{12}, and folate deficiency
bruising	areas of skin that are blue/black in colour	in CRF, the bleeding time is increased, leading to bleeding in tissues
pigmentation	areas of darkened skin on either the face or limbs; pale yellow tinge to skin	increased production of melanin-stimulating hormone causes melanin deposition in the skin; also, urochrome deposition in the skin

Fig. 7.2 Signs related to skin colour in renal disease. (CRF, chronic renal failure.)

Signs in the face & neck related to renal disease		
Test	**Sign**	**Diagnostic inference**
polycythaemia	red and rugged appearance of the face	occasionally seen in: • polycystic kidneys • post-transplant • carcinoma of the kidney
uraemic frost	white powdery crystals of urate look like dandruff on the forehead	the crystals form from excess urea in the sweat and are a terminal sign of CRF
deposits in the sclera	yellow deposits in the sclera	calcium deposits due to hyperparathyroidism
retinal changes		seen in: • diabetes mellitus • hypertension • vascular disease
ear function	deafness	Alport syndrome
ulcers	ulceration of the mouth and lips	severely ill patients (impaired immune system)
fungal infection	white deposit in the mouth	patients on cytotoxic drugs or steroids; immunosuppression with drugs can result in opportunistic infections such as candidal infection
halitosis (bad breath)	• ammonia smell • acetone smell	• renal failure • ketoacidosis

Fig. 7.3 Signs in the face & neck related to renal disease. (CRF, chronic renal failure.)

Respiratory signs seen in renal disease		
Test	**Sign**	**Diagnostic inference**
observe the pattern and rate of respiration	deep sighing breathing with rapid respiratory rate (Kussmaul's respiration)	• systemic acidosis causes direct stimulation of the respiratory centre: seen in uraemia due to the retention of H^+ • a similar respiratory pattern is observed in severe untreated diabetic ketoacidosis

Fig. 7.4 Respiratory signs in renal disease.

Signs related to dialysis equipment		
Test	**Sign**	**Diagnostic inference**
observe equipment around the patient and on the adjacent table	• dialysis machine • fistula • CAPD catheter	acute or end-stage renal failure requiring dialysis

Fig. 7.5 Signs related to dialysis equipment. (CAPD, continuous ambulatory peritoneal dialysis).

○ **List what you should do before you start to examine a patient.**
○ **List features you might observe that can help you in making a clinical assessment of the patient.**

HANDS AND LIMBS

The signs on the hands and nails that are indicative of underlying renal disease are shown in Fig. 7.6. Fig. 7.7 shows the finger signs seen in renal disease, while changes in the limbs in renal disease are listed in Fig. 7.8.

○ **What hand signs may be observed in renal disease?**

Nail signs in renal disease		
Test	**Sign**	**Diagnostic inference**
markings on nail	transverse ridges (Beau's lines)	indicative of: • past malnutrition • severe illness
	splinter haemorrhages	renal failure due to: • vasculitis (e.g. Wegener's granulomatosis) • bacterial endocarditis
discoloration of nails	brown discoloration of nails	CRF
	opaque white discoloration of the nails	nephrotic syndrome and CRF

Fig. 7.6 Nail signs in renal disease. (CRF, chronic renal failure.)

Finger signs in renal disease		
Test	**Sign**	**Diagnostic inference**
examine the fingers spread out on a flat surface to assess any changes in length	shortening of the distal phalanges, resulting in a difference of length between the fingers of right and left hands	typical finding in severe renal osteodystrophy secondary to CRF due to chronic high levels of parathyroid hormone
ask patients to hold hands straight out in front of them and watch for any movement; a piece of paper can be put on top of the hands to ease detection of any movement	a coarse dipping movement is seen in the outstretched fingers and is exaggerated by dorsiflexing the wrists	• severe uraemia: a preterminal sign in patients with renal disease indicating the need for immediate renal replacement therapy; indistinguishable from any of the other metabolic flaps (asterixis) due to: • CO_2 retention in respiratory failure • chronic liver disease

Fig. 7.7 Finger signs in renal disease.

Changes in the limbs in renal disease		
Test	**Sign**	**Diagnostic inference**
appearance and texture of skin	dry flaky skin	CRF
	scratch marks and bruises on limbs and abdomen	uraemic pruritus due to hyperphosphataemia and dry skin
	dirty brown appearance which can make the patient look very healthy	CRF causing an increase in photosensitive pigment (pseudoporphyrin) as a result of decreased clearance of porphyrins in the urine and increased melanin secondary to increased MSH
skin scars or lesions	fistulae are often seen on the forearm	allow access to blood at a high pressure for haemodialysis
	scars from previous surgically constructed fistulae	vascular access clots and often needs reconstruction
deformities of bones and joints; check range of movement, signs of inflammation and for any pain	valgus (knock knees) and varus (bow legs) deformities	renal rickets due to renal osteodystrophy
	painful, inflamed and red	acute gout due to the deposition of urate crystals in joints
look for any involuntary movement	sporadic twitching of limbs (often accompanies a tremor)	indicative of need for immediate renal replacement therapy
	some patients have an uncontrollable need to move their limbs all the time (restless limbs)	CRF or on dialysis
measure blood pressure	postural drop in BP	hypovolaemia
oedema: pitting if there is indentation of the skin after 10 s of finger pressure	generalized swelling of limb and pitting; if present at ankle, check at knee and mid-thigh	pitting oedema is characteristic of: • fluid overload due to salt and water retention • nephrotic syndrome • congestive cardiac failure
rash	purpuric rash (cutaneous haemorrhage)	vasculitis (e.g. Henoch–Schönlein purpura)
skin and subcutaneous tissue turgor: assessed by rolling a pinch of soft tissue between finger and thumb	the skin will seem less elastic and tense	skin and subcutaneous turgor is reduced in: • old age • Na+ depletion • malnutrition
peripheral neuropathy	a glove and stocking distribution of peripheral sensory loss	advanced renal failure (rare)

Fig. 7.8 Changes in the limbs in renal disease. (CRF, chronic renal failure.)

THORAX

Respiratory system

Very little is seen in the respiratory examination related to renal disease. Hyperventilation and Kussmaul's respiration are seen with the acidosis of advanced CRF (Fig. 7.4).

Cardiovascular system (CVS)
Blood pressure (BP)

This is very important in renal disease since many patients will have an elevated BP. When monitoring BP on various occasions it is important to measure it on the same limb each time to ensure consistent and comparable results. To ensure accurate measurement the correct cuff size must be used on a fully extended arm with the stethoscope applied lightly to the brachial artery. The BP should always be taken lying and sitting down, and standing because:

- The increase in diastolic pressure on standing of 5–10 mmHg indicates a healthy CVS.
- Postural hypotension is only detected if both measurements are taken.

The World Health Organization (WHO) definition for hypertension is a maintained diastolic pressure of over 90 mmHg. The renal diseases associated with hypertension include renal artery stenosis, acute and chronic glomerulonephritis (GN), polycystic kidneys, and nephrotic syndrome.

Observation, palpation, percussion, and auscultation

Examination of the CVS is done with the patient sitting up at 45° and undressed from the waist up. Ensure the patient is comfortable. Fig. 7.9 shows general findings in the CVS in renal disease, while Fig. 7.10 shows the findings on palpation in the CVS examination. The positive findings on percussion and auscultation of the CVS are respectively shown in Figs 7.11 and 7.12.

General findings in the cardiovascular system in renal disease		
Test	**Sign**	**Diagnostic inference**
abnormality of chest wall	increased curvature of spine and rounded shoulders	softening of vertebrae due to renal osteodystrophy in the spine (rugger jersey spine on radiograph)
scars: note position on chest and check round to back following the ribs	midline scars	previous heart surgery
	old scars are white and pale and recent scars are purple–red in colour	
jugular venous pressure (an indicator of internal fluid load): the patient should be at 45° and with head turned away from you; note any pulsations in the internal jugular vein	normally jugular venous pulse is not visible, but can be seen by occluding the vein just above the clavicle	jugular venous pressure is raised in: • right heart failure • fluid overload • chronic bronchitis
	if a waveform is visible then measure the height from the top of the fluid level vertically down to the angle of Louis	

Fig. 7.9 General findings in the cardiovascular system in renal disease.

Findings on palpation in the cardiovascular system examination in renal disease		
Test	**Sign**	**Diagnostic inference**
apex beat is normally felt in the mid-clavicular line at the level of the fifth intercostal space; this is the most lateral point at which the pulsation can be felt—note its position and strength	lateral displacement	left ventricular dilatation causing enlargement of the heart pneumothorax
	impalpable	• obesity • pleural effusion • pericardial effusion
	thrusting and strong	• high blood pressure • left ventricular hypertrophy
peripheral pulses	presence or absence listen with a stethoscope for bruits	atherosclerosis if present may suggest renovascular disease

Fig. 7.10 Findings on palpation on examination of the cardiovascular system in renal disease.

Positive findings on percussion of the cardiovascular system in renal disease		
Test	**Sign**	**Diagnostic inference**
heart borders	dull to percussion beyond the normal boundaries of the mediastinum	enlargement of heart
bases of lungs	decreased breath sounds	pleural effusion in: • nephrotic syndrome • congestive cardiac failure • fluid retention

Fig. 7.11 Positive findings on percussion of the cardiovascular system in renal disease.

Positive findings on auscultation of the cardiovascular system in renal disease		
Test	**Sign**	**Diagnostic inference**
heart sounds: listen for audibility, rate and accentuation of the sound in all four areas	muffled and soft	pericardial effusion
	prominent aortic component of the second heart sound	hypertension
	a low-pitched third heart sound heard after the second heart sound	an early sign of left ventricular failure or fluid overload
	gallop rhythm (two normal heart sounds with a third and tachycardia)	• fluid overload • ventricular failure
murmurs: • low pitch (apex) with the bell • high pitch with the diaphragm feel the carotid pulse—time the murmur with the cardiac cycle	• functional murmurs • murmurs due to coexisting valve disease	• aortic and pulmonary regurgitation due to dilatation of the valve ring secondary to fluid overload • mitral regurgitation due to annular calification of the valve; anaemia
pericardial rub: listen carefully over the precordium	a localized or generalized scratchy sound heard in any part of the cardiac cycle heard best if the patient leans forward	this friction rub (two layers of the pericardial layer moving in the presence of an exudate) occurs in: • pericarditis (a terminal feature of CRF) • uraemic pericarditis • systemic lupus erythematosus and vasculitis • intermittent illness in a patient with CRF

Fig. 7.12 Positive findings on auscultation of the cardiovascular system in renal disease. (CRF, chronic renal failure.)

- **What measures should you take to obtain consistent and comparable blood pressure measurements?**
- **List possible CVS findings on palpation, percussion, and auscultation in renal disease.**

ABDOMEN

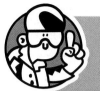

Overview

General points of the clinical examination are discussed earlier in the chapter. The patient should be lying as flat as possible on a firm mattress with arms by the side and head supported with one or two pillows—check that the patient is comfortable. This position ensures that the abdominal muscles are relaxed, making palpation much easier.

Stand on the right hand side of the bed, ideally with the patient exposed from 'nipples to knees'; to maintain privacy expose the patient from the xiphisternum to the level of the symphysis pubis.

Examination of the genitalia is a vital part of examination of the abdominal system. They should either be covered up once inspection is complete or be examined later.

Observation

This is a vital part of the examination and it is worth spending 20–30 s just looking at the patient from the end of the bed. Look around the patient for any clues—

In an exam say that you would go on to examine the genitalia and if necessary perform a rectal examination once you have completed the abdominal examination.

drips, drains, and dialysis machines. Fig. 7.13 shows the signs usually seen on general inspection of the abdomen in a patient with renal disease.

Palpation

Before you start to palpate ask patients whether they are in pain and ask them to point to the painful or tender area. Your should start palpating from the point furthest from the locus of the pain. Tell the patient to breathe normally and relax—you will be able to feel much more through relaxed abdominal muscles. It may help to kneel at the bedside so that you are at the same

Signs on general inspection of the abdomen in renal disease		
Test	**Sign**	**Diagnostic inference**
abnormality of the abdominal contours:		renal causes of a distended abdomen are: • fluid (ascites or CAPD fluid)
• general distension	• general fullness and enlargement of the abdominal cavity • the skin of the abdomen is shiny and smooth	other (nonrenal) causes include: • fat • flatus • fetus • faeces (constipation)
• localized distension observe to see if abdomen moves with or independently of respiration	symmetrical swelling	polycystic kidneys
	asymmetrical swelling	enlarged kidney; kidney transplant in the iliac regions
scars: note position on the abdomen and check round to the back following the ribs to the spine	midline scars	previous abdominal surgery
	iliac scars overlying a mass	kidney transplants
	lateral longitudinal scars extending around the back	nephrectomy scars
	note that old scars are white and pale and recent scars are purple–red in colour	

Fig. 7.13 Signs on general inspection of the abdomen in renal disease.

Remember the causes of a
distended abdomen as the 5 Fs:
- **Fat**
- **Fluid**
- **Flatus**
- **Fetus**
- **Faeces**

level as the patient and this is important to demonstrate in an examination.

Have a routine for examining all the regions and organs to avoid missing anything out:

1. Begin with gentle palpation of the nine regions of the abdomen; then repeat using deeper palpation—keep looking at the patient's face for any signs of discomfort.
2. Then examine the liver and spleen while the patient is breathing deeply in and out.
3. Next examine the kidneys and urinary bladder, feel for the aorta, and then check the hernial orifices while asking the patient to cough.
4. If you feel any mass there are certain characteristics you must define about it—these are site, size, shape, edge, surface (regular or irregular), consistency, mobility, movement with respiration, whether it is pulsatile and resonance to percussion also check for associated scars and listen over it for a bruit.
5. Remember to tell the patient that you need to examine the genitalia.

Fig. 7.14 explains how the kidneys are examined and shows relevant findings in various renal conditions.

How the kidneys are examined and relevant findings in various renal conditions		
Test	**Sign**	**Diagnostic inference**
bimanual examination of the kidneys: • place the right hand anteriorly in the lumbar region and the left hand posteriorly under the patient in the loin • push up with the left hand as the patient takes a deep breath in • ballot the kidneys between both hands (i.e. push the kidney from one hand to the other) • repeat on the other side keeping the right hand anterior	the kidney is normally impalpable (except in very thin people) and if easily felt suggests an abnormality the lower pole is felt as a firm round edge between both hands on deep inspiration (it must be distinguished from an enlarged liver or spleen) there is minimal movement on respiration an irregular kidney surface felt in polycystic disease	unilateral enlargement: • tumour • renal cyst • hydronephrosis • compensatory hypertrophy bilateral enlargement: • polycystic kidneys • hydronephrosis • tumour (rare)
examination of the urinary bladder: • the bladder is palpated from the umbilicus down to the symphysis pubis • the upper and lateral borders are easily felt • the inferior border is impalpable	not normally palpable when enlarged it is felt as a smooth rounded firm cystic mass in the suprapubic region it is not always symmetrical and in the midline	chronic retention of urine acute retention is associated with bladder tenderness distended bladders are not always palpable in obesity
pain: • check carefully if the patient is in pain • the nature of the pain is important in determining the site of the lesion • assess pain by asking the patient to point to the pain and asking what the pain is like	fixed constant pain; colicky pain superimposed on a constant dull pain	kidney pain
	radiation of pain from the flank to the groin and iliac fossa; the patient is usually writhing in pain and is doubled up	ureteric distension due to obstruction in the ureters, most commonly renal stones as they are passed down the ureter

Fig. 7.14 How to examine the kidneys and relevant findings in a variety of renal conditions.

Percussion

Percussion in the abdomen is used to elicit the cause of any distension and the composition of any mass—fluid-filled cysts and solid tumours are dull to percussion. Fig. 7.15 shows the findings observed on percussion of the abdomen in patients with renal disease.

Auscultation

Fig. 7.16 shows the findings on auscultation of the abdomen in renal disease.

Rectal examination

Fig. 7.17 shows the findings on rectal examination in renal disease.

Findings observed on percussion of the abdomen in renal disease		
Test	**Sign**	**Diagnostic inference**
ascites (excess free fluid in the peritoneal cavity): • presence shown by shifting of dullness • the abdomen is percussed from the flank into the midline for any areas of dullness • keep your hand on the area of dullness • ask the patient to roll away from you on to his or her side • percuss in this area with the patient in the new position and see if it is now resonant to percussion • this can be confirmed by asking the patient to roll over onto the other side	positive shifting dullness is indicative of ascites the area that was previously dull to percussion becomes resonant due to redistribution of fluid in the peritoneal cavity	causes of ascites in renal disease: • nephrotic syndrome • peritoneal dialysis • idiopathic ascites of dialysis • perineal dialysis fluid
percussion of the bladder: always percuss from above the umbilicus down to the pubic bone	resonance followed by dullness consistent with an enlarged cystic mass	distension of the urinary bladder due to chronic or acute retention

Fig. 7.15 Findings on percussion of the abdomen in renal disease.

Findings on auscultation in renal disease		
Test	**Sign**	**Diagnostic inference**
bruits: listen for these by applying the stethoscope firmly on a relaxed abdomen or in the flank over the renal artery; they may also be listened for over the back	rapid and turbulent movement of blood through a narrowed vessel	• renal artery stenosis • atherosclerosis • arteriovenous malformation in the kidney it can be difficult to determine whether the bruit originates in the aorta or renal artery

Fig. 7.16 Findings on auscultation in renal disease.

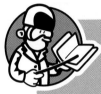

Fig. 7.17 Findings on rectal examination in renal disease.

Findings on rectal examination in renal disease		
Test	Sign	Diagnostic inference
digital examination of the rectum—vital for a complete abdominal (see *Crash Course: Gastrointestinal System*) and urological examination	firm and smooth with a rubbery feel	normal prostate
the prostate is felt with the patient in the left lateral position	tender, enlarged and soft	acute infection (prostatitis)
	hard and irregular	carcinoma of the prostate

○ **What measures should you take to carry out an abdominal examination?**
○ **Describe in order the steps for palpating the abdomen.**
○ **List possible findings on palpation, percussion, and auscultation of the abdomen in renal disease.**

INVESTIGATIVE TECHNIQUES

Imaging is a very useful investigation in renal disease when used in conjunction with other investigative techniques (Figs 8.1–8.3). Radiological imaging of the kidney and urinary tract may allow a diagnosis to be established, assessment of the complications of impaired renal function, and monitoring of the progression of disease or the response to therapy.

Ultrasonography

Ultrasonography is an inexpensive and non-invasive technique that is used to asses the size, shape and position of the kidney. It can also detect space-occupying lesions and is ideal for screening relatives of patients with polycystic disease (Figs 8.4 and 8.5). Enlargement of the prostate can also be assessed, and this can further be investigated with the use of transurethral ultrasonography as guidance for prostatic biopsy (Fig. 8.6). Renal vein thrombosis can be detected with Doppler ultrasonography.

Plain radiography

Plain radiography of the kidney, ureters, and bladder is a simple, noninvasive test that can be used before specialized imaging. It is used to detect calcification in the kidney, such as renal and urinary tract stones—uric acid stones cannot be detected, but in general 90% of stones are radio-opaque (Figs 8.7–8.9).

Microbiological test results and their significance				
	Indications	Scientific basis	Normal results	Abnormal results
urine culture	must always be performed if UTI symptoms or any renal disease is suspected; in cases of TB an early morning sample of urine is required	growing any organisms present; vital to have an MSU specimen	no growth	>100 000 CFU/mL indicates urinary infection < 10 000 CFU/mL probably indicates contamination of the specimen
antibodies (i) streptococcal Ag	suspicion of past streptococcal glomerulonephritis	antibodies are made in response to infection and may trigger glomerulonephritis		increased titres of: AntiDNAase B ASOT consistent with poststreptococcal glomerulonephrits
(ii) hepatitis	renal disease associated with liver disease	infection with hepatits B and C have effects on the kidney		hepatitis B causes polyarteritis nodosa membranous nephropathy hepatitis C causes cryoglobulinaemia
(iii) HIV	patients at risk of HIV with renal symptoms	infection with HIV can cause renal damage		HIV-associated glomerulonephritis
malaria	those who have recently returned from the tropics and have recurrent fevers			ring-form parasites observed on peripheral blood film

Fig. 8.1 Microbiological tests and their significance (ASOT, antistreptococcal O antigen titre; CFU, colony-forming units; MSU, mid-stream urine.)

Blood test results and their significance				
	Indications	**Scientific basis**	**Normal results**	**Abnormal results**
urea	oligouria & anuria; dehydration; hypertension; diabetes mellitus; oedema; nausea & vomiting; loin pain	crude indication of renal function	2.5–6.6 mmol/L	increased in: renal disease; high protein intake; fever; gastrointestinal haemorrhage
creatinine	same as above for urea	reciprocal relationship with GFR—reflects renal function	62–124 mmol/L	increased in all types of renal disease; N.B. GFR may fall by 50% before urea or creatinine go outside the reference range
albumin	oedema	gives an assessment of severity of urinary protein losses in proteinuria	35–50 g/L	hypoalbuminaemia nephrotic syndome hyperalbuminaemia dehydration
sodium, potassium, anion gap	confusion; lethargy; seizures; coma; arrythmias; hypertension; hypotension; tachycardia/bradycardia; vomiting; diarrhoea; heavy sweating; diabetes mellitus; polyuria; polydipsia	changes in the concentration of sodium, potassium and the anion gap are found in renal diseases; potassium is important in the function of excitable tissues and is important for survival	Na=135–145 mmol/L K=3.5–5.0 mmol/L anion gap = 8–16 mmol/L	hypernatraemia hyponatraemia hyperkalaemia hypokalaemia increased anion gap in: renal failure ketoacidosis (diabetes melitus) hyperlactaemia (from shock) anion ingestion
arterial blood gases and pH (uses arterial blood)	hypoperfusion; hyperventilation; Kussmaul's breathing in diabetic ketoacidosis; ingestion of acids; diarrhoea; vomiting	oxygen concentration is important as it reflects tissue perfusion; an increase in CO_2 is lethal and poisonous to cells; pH is vital because most cells in the body work at an optimal pH and are very sensitive to changes in pH	$pO_2 = 10.6–13.0$ kPa $pCO_2 = 4.7–6.0$ kPa pH = 7.35–7.45	acidosis commonly found in renal failure; compensated for by respiratory stimulation $\downarrow pCO_2$
haemoglobin	chronic renal failure; haemorrhage	the haemoglobin levels are important as Hb carries oxygen to the tissues.	male 13.5–18.0 g/dL female 11.5–16.0 g/dL	decreased Hb chronic renal failure blood loss polycythaemia renal tumours renal cysts
ESR	loin pain; symptoms of UTI; systemic disease		<15 mm/h	increased in infection renal cell carcinoma retroperitoneal fibrosis vasculitis
PSA (prostate-specific antigen)	any men aged >45 years with prostatism or UTIs	the level of PSA increases with prostatic cancer and metastatic disease; used to monitor therapy success		increased in prostatic carcinoma silent recurrence of carcinoma metastatic disease small increase in prostatic hyperplasia
urate	kidney stones; patients with large tumour loads given chemotherapy; 'tumour lysis' syndrome → urate	hyperuricaemia can cause urate deposition in renal tract	0.12–0.42 mmol/L	increased in gout renal and urinary calculi
calcium	kidney stones; myeloma; metastatic disease	hypercalcaemia causes calcium deposition in renal tract; hypercalcuria also causes urinary concentrating defects	2.0–2.6 mmol/L	increased in renal and urinary calculi

Fig. 8.2 Blood test results and their significance.

		Urine biochemistry test results and their significance		
	Indications	**Scientific basis**	**Normal results**	**Abnormal results**
appearance	any urine sample		clear fluid	**red/pink:** haematuria, beetroot intake **brown:** concentrated cholestatic jaundice **cloudy:** infection
volume	any urine sample		1000–2500 mL/day	**oliguria:** physiological; intrinsic renal disease; obstructive nephropathy **polyuria:** excess H_2O intake; increased solute loss e.g. glucose; concentration failure
pH	any urine sample		pH 4.5–8.0	**alkaline urine:** infection with *Proteus*—urea splitting **acid urine:** aminoaciduria; renal calculi
sodium	oliguria altered Na^+ homeostasis	urinary [Na] must be interpreted in context of urine output, sodium intake and natriuretic drugs	depends on clinical setting; 24-hour urinary Na^+ = 100–250 mmol/L	<20 mmol/L oliguria minoaciduria; renal calculi <20 mmol/L oliguria →prerenal <20 mmol/L and not oliguric →extrarenal losses >20 mmol/L renal losses
creatinine and creatinine clearance	similar to those for blood creatinine levels	creatinine clearance reflects GFR; both the urine and plasma concentration of creatinine is required; requires timed urine collection	125 mL/min per 1.73 m^2 body surface area	decreased levels indicate a decrease in GFR—as see in acute and chronic renal diseases
blood	gross bleeding into urine usually found in patients with renal disease; hypertension; pregnancy; bacterial endocarditis	reagent strips are used—based on a peroxide-like reaction	nil any positive result must be followed by microscopy	**microscopic haematuria:** renal disease, i.e. nephritic syndrome; blood at the beginning of voiding then clear—from the urethra; blood throughout voiding—from the bladder or above; blood only at the end of voiding—from the prostate or base of the bladder
protein dipstick and if positive → 24-hour collection	oedema	reagent strips impregnated with buffered blue tetrabromophenol—detects [albumin] >150 mg/L; microalbuminuria is used as an earlier indicator of diabetic glomerular disease; the test requires a radioimmunoassay ↑ which is more sensitive than the strips	<150 mg /day random sample = < 100 mg/L (>0.3g/L is detected on the sticks) microalbuminuria = 30–150 μg/min or 0.2–2.8 mg/mmol of protein	**increased with:** exercise; standing up; renal disease; nephrotic syndrome; fever; diabetic glomerular disease; hypertension
glucose	suspected diabetes mellitus; renal disease; pregnancy	reagent strips using glucose oxidase or hexokinase enzyme reactions Clinitest	nil	glucose may be present when: 1. blood glucose above the renal threshold i.e. diabetes mellitus 2. altered renal threshold i.e. pregnancy; renal disease
urine microscopy (obtain a clean urine sample i.e. MSU) **(i) direct** **(ii) after centrifugation**	symptoms of UTIs; suspicion of renal disease	a small amount of unspun urine placed on a slide, covered with a cover slip and looked at under a microscope. Gram stain to look for bacteria counterstained to look at cell cytology	nil	**white cells indicate:** inflammatory reaction; infection in the urinary tract; stones; TB; analgesic nephropathy **red cells indicate:** glomrulonephritis; acute urinary tract infection; calculi; tumour **granular casts indicate:** acute tubular necrosis; rapidly progressing glomerulonephritis **white blood cell casts indicate:** pyelonephritis **red cell casts indicate:** glomerulonephritis **crystals seen indicate:** stones **bacteria seen indicate:** infection **abnormal cells indicate:** cancer of urothelium

Fig. 8.3 Urine test results and their significance.

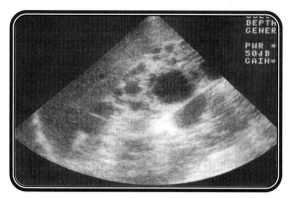

Fig. 8.4 Ultrasound scan showing the typical appearance of polycystic kidneys. There are multiple cysts within the parenchyma. (From Color Atlas of Urology 2e by Dr RW Lloyd-Davis, Dr H Parkhouse, Dr JG Gow, and Dr DR Davies. Mosby Year Book. 1994.)

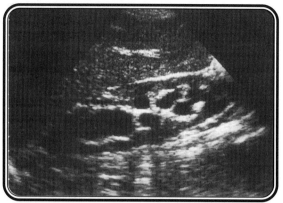

Fig. 8.5 Hydronephrosis of the right kidney demonstrated by ultrasonography. The echo-lucent (black) areas within the kidney are caused by dilated calyces. (From Color Atlas of Renal Diseases 2e, by Dr G Williams and Professor NP Mallick. Mosby Year Book, 1994.)

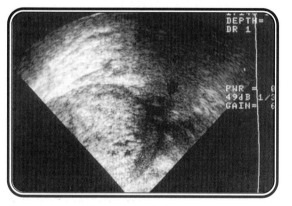

Fig. 8.6 A rectal ultrasound probe is used to define and stage carcinoma of the prostate. An echo-poor area in the left peripheral zone of the prostate is extending into the central part of the gland and beyond the capsule of the gland (arrow). (Courtesy of Dr D Rickards.)

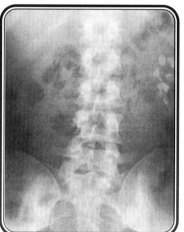

Fig. 8.7 This plain abdominal radiograph shows calculi occupying most of the left kidney. (Courtesy of Mr RS Cole.)

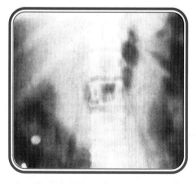

Fig. 8.8 This plain abdominal radiograph shows a single calyceal calculus in a patient who presented with renal colic. (From Color Atlas of Urology 2e by Dr RW Lloyd-Davis, Dr H Parkhouse, Dr JG Gow, and Dr DR Davies. Mosby Year Book. 1994.)

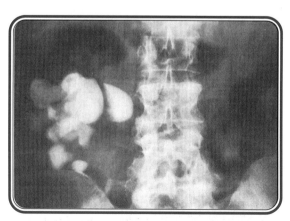

Fig. 8.9 This plain abdominal radiograph shows a large staghorn calculus in the right kidney in a patient who presented with recurrent urinary tract infections. (From Color Atlas of Renal Diseases 2e, by Dr G Williams and Professor NP Mallick. Mosby Year Book, 1994.)

Biopsy

Renal biopsy is used to classify glomerulonephritis and therefore predict response to steroid treatment in patients with nephrotic syndrome. It is also used in the diagnosis and assessment of systemic lupus erythematosus. It may aid the investigation of unexplained acute renal failure, proteinuria, and haematuria. It is vital in the management of renal transplant patients. A specimen of the kidney can be taken by inserting a needle into the back guided by ultrasound.

Intravenous urography and intravenous pyelography

Intravenous urography (IVU) and pyelography (IVP) involve serial films taken after injection of radio-opaque contrast medium (Figs 8.10–8.13). These techniques are used to assess renal size and outline and the architecture and patency of the calyces and pelvis.

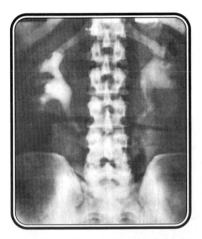

Fig. 8.10 In this case, there is bilateral hydronephrosis typical of retroperitoneal fibrosis. An intravenous urogram is the gold-standard investigation in acute renal colic. (From *Color Atlas of Urology* 2e by Dr RW Lloyd-Davis, Dr H Parkhouse, Dr JG Gow, and Dr DR Davies. Mosby Year Book. 1994.)

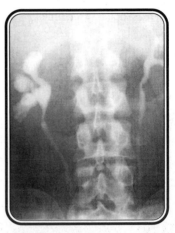

Fig. 8.11 An intravenous urogram showing marked calyceal clubbing in the right kidney. There is gross dilatation of the calyces, which is pronounced in all poles of the kidney. These findings are the result of unilateral reflux of urine and chronic infection. (From *Color Atlas of Urology* 2e by Dr RW Lloyd-Davis, Dr H Parkhouse, Dr JG Gow, and Dr DR Davies. Mosby Year Book. 1994.)

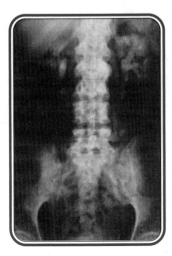

Fig. 8.12 An intravenous urogram demonstrating two small contracted kidneys. There is cortical scarring and calyceal dilatation and deformity. These features are characteristic of reflux nephropathy (chronic pyelonephritis). (From *Color Atlas of Urology* 2e by Dr RW Lloyd-Davis, Dr H Parkhouse, Dr JG Gow, and Dr DR Davies. Mosby Year Book. 1994.)

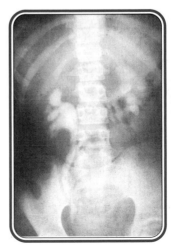

Fig. 8.13 An intravenous urogram showing bilateral hydronephrosis in response to bladder neck obstruction caused by dense granulation and fibrous tissue in a patient with schistosomiasis of the bladder. (From *Color Atlas of Renal Diseases* 2e, by Dr G Williams and Professor NP Mallick. Mosby Year Book, 1994.)

Renal arteriography

Renal arteriography gives an anatomical demonstration of the renal arteries. It is used to detect renal artery stenosis or aneurysms (Figs 8.14 and 8.15). It can be used in the diagnosis of tumours, but this is becoming less common with the increasing use of CT. Contrast is injected into the renal artery through a catheter introduced into the femoral artery and a series of radiographs are taken.

Micturating cystourethrography

Micturating cystourethrograms are used to demonstrate vesicoureteric reflux from the bladder to the ureters during emptying of the bladder (Fig. 8.16). Reflux can be classified according to three grades.

- Grade 1—contrast medium enters the ureter only.
- Grade 2—contrast medium fills the pelvicalyceal system.

- Grade 3—dilatation of the calyces and ureter.

This technique is used to investigate children with recurrent urinary tract infections and adults with disturbed bladder function.

Cystoscopy

A rigid or flexible cystoscope can be used to inspect the interior of the bladder and urethra. This technique is very useful in the diagnosis and treatment of tumours in the bladder. It can also be used in the assessment of prostatic disease.

Retrograde pyelography

Retrograde pyelography is used to define the site of an obstruction (Figs 8.17 and 8.18) or lesions within the ureter. It involves cystoscopy of a catheterized patient

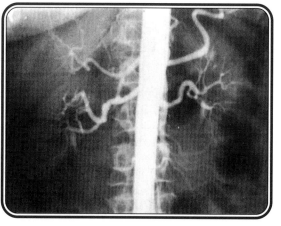

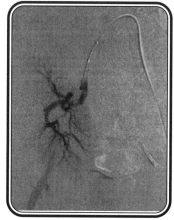

Fig. 8.15 Subtraction arteriogram of a transplanted kidney. The donor renal artery is anastamosed to the internal iliac artery. (From Color Atlas of Renal Diseases 2e, by Dr G Williams and Professor NP Mallick. Mosby Year Book, 1994.)

Fig. 8.14 An arteriogram showing renal artery stenosis. The stenosis is marked on the right and is typical of stenosis caused by fibromuscular hyperplasia. (From Color Atlas of Renal Diseases 2e, by Dr G Williams and Professor NP Mallick. Mosby Year Book, 1994.)

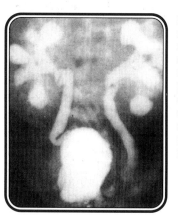

Fig. 8.16 A micturating cystourethrogram showing bilateral ureteric reflux. This patient has early calyceal clubbing and ureteric dilatation (grade-3 reflux). (Courtesy of RS Cole.)

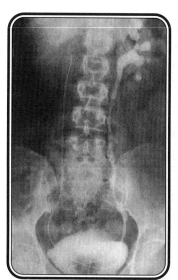

Fig. 8.17 Retrograde pyelogram showing emphysematous pyelonephritis caused by gas-forming bacteria. (From Diagnostic Picture Tests in Renal Disease, by Professor GRD Catto, Dr PAJ Brown, and Dr IH Khan. TMIP. 1994.)

and contrast is used to define the lesions.

Computed tomography

Computed tomography (CT) is useful in defining renal and retroperitoneal masses and is especially useful in locating and staging renal tumours (Fig. 8.19). It is also used to show polycystic kidney disease. Modern techniques involving spiral CT can be used to visualize the anatomy of the renal arteries, renal vein, and inferior vena cava.

Radionuclide scanning

Radionuclide scans are used in static and dynamic imaging. Technetium-labelled dimercaptosuccinic acid (^{99m}Tc-DMSA) provides images of the renal parenchyma, and will show scarring as a result of reflux nephropathy (Fig. 8.20), whereas technetium-labelled pentetic acid

(^{99m}Tc-DTPA) gives information about the vascularity of the kidneys. It is used in the assessment of transplant function (Fig. 8.21) and can demonstrate obstruction to the upper urinary tract (by diuresis renogram).

Urodynamic studies

These are used to distinguish urge incontinence from stress incontinence. It also detects bladder/detrusor muscle instability. The bladder is catheterized and a pressure probe is inserted to measure the bladder pressure. A rectal probe is also inserted to assess intra-abdominal pressure. The bladder is then filled with water until the patient feels the urge to void. At this point the relative pressures are recorded.

Other imaging techniques

Other imaging techniques include scintigraphy (Fig. 8.22).

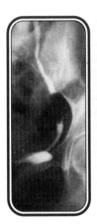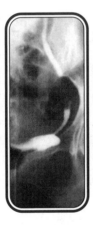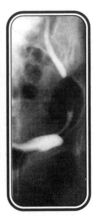

Fig. 8.18 Retrograde pyelogram showing a large filling defect in the left ureter caused by a tumour. (From *Color Atlas of Urology* 2e by Dr RW Lloyd-Davis, Dr H Parkhouse, Dr JG Gow, and Dr DR Davies. Mosby Year Book. 1994.)

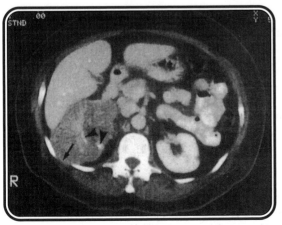

Fig. 8.19 CT scan demonstrating a right renal cell carcinoma that extends through the intercostal space between ribs 11 and 12 (arrow) and medially along the renal vein. The high attenuation (white) areas (arrowheads) in the lesion are caused by calcification. (From *Color Atlas of Renal Diseases* 2e, by Dr G Williams and Professor NP Mallick. Mosby Year Book, 1994.)

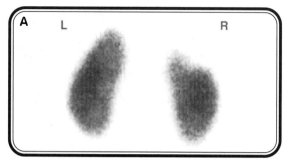

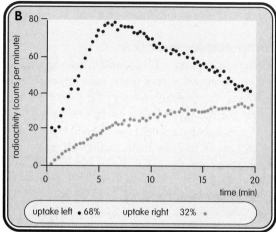

Fig. 8.20 (A) ^{99m}Tc-DMSA scan showing a right upper pole scar. (Courtesy of TO Nunan.) (B) The graph shows a diminution of uptake of 36% for the right kidney, indicating a similar degree of loss of function. (From Color Atlas of Renal Diseases 2e, by Dr G Williams and Professor NP Mallick. Mosby Year Book, 1994.)

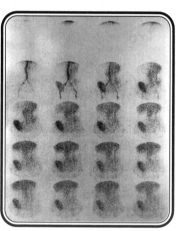

Fig. 8.21 ^{99m}Tc-DTPA diuretic renogram showing a transplanted kidney functioning normally. (From Diagnostic Picture Tests in Renal Disease, by Professor GRD Catto, Dr PAJ Brown, and Dr IH Khan. TMIP. 1994.)

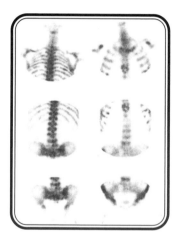

Fig. 8.22 This bone scintigram shows multiple bone metastases in a patient with carcinoma of the prostate. There are areas of increased activity in the ribs, sternum, and pelvis. (Courtesy of Dr TO Nunan.)

- Explain the indications for the following investigations, indicate on whom the test is performed, state what would be a normal result and discuss the interpretation of abnormal results for the following:
  - Blood tests (urea, creatinine, albumin, sodium, potassium, anion gap, arterial blood gases and pH, and haemoglobin).
  - Urine tests (sodium, creatinine and creatinine clearance, blood, protein, glucose, microscopy, culture and cytology).
  - Imaging of the kidney (ultrasonography, plain radiography, intravenous pyelography, micturating cystourethrography, retrograde pyelography, renal arteriography, cystoscopy and urodynamic studies).
- What are the indications for a renal biopsy and how is it performed?
- What abnormalities may be found?

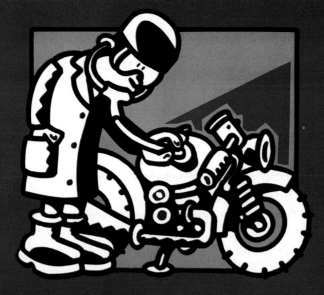

BASIC PATHOLOGY

CONGENITAL ABNORMALITIES OF THE KIDNEY

Various congenital structural abnormalities can be observed within the kidney and these are described below.

Agenesis of the kidney

Absence of the kidney can be either bilateral or unilateral. Bilateral agenesis occurs in about 0.04% of all pregnancies and is not compatible with life. It is also known as Potter's syndrome and is associated with pulmonary hypoplasia. There is oligohydramnios *in utero*.

Unilateral agenesis

This condition occurs in 1 in 1000 of the population. The only kidney present becomes hypertrophied, but tends to be abnormal with malrotation, ectopia or hydronephrosis. The kidney is at risk of infection and trauma. This disorder is associated with other developmental abnormalities such as spina bifida, meningomyelocoele and congenital heart disease.

Hypoplasia

The kidneys fail to develop adequately and are consequently smaller than average. One or both kidneys can be affected. This disorder is rare and the kidneys are prone to infection and stone formation.

Ectopic kidney

The incidence of ectopic kidney is 1 in 800. The kidney is found in an abnormal site (usually the pelvis—therefore sometimes called 'pelvic kidney') (Fig. 9.1). It presents as a pelvic mass. Due to the abnormal positioning, the ureters can be obstructed by neighbouring structures, resulting in obstructive uropathy, infection, and stone formation. This disorder may also interfere with parturition.

Horseshoe kidney

The incidence of horseshoe kidney is between 1 in 600 and 1 in 1800. The two kidneys become fused across the midline, usually at their lower poles (Fig. 9.2). The kidneys are usually joined by renal tissue or a fibrous band. The horseshoe kidney is usually lower than normal because the inferior mesenteric artery limits its ascent. It may also be malrotated and is prone to reflux, obstruction, infection, and stone formation.

Fig. 9.1 Ectopic (pelvic) kidney.

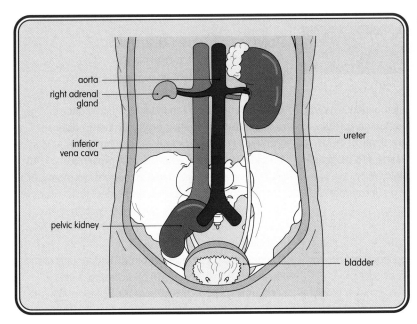

aorta
right adrenal gland
inferior vena cava
pelvic kidney
ureter
bladder

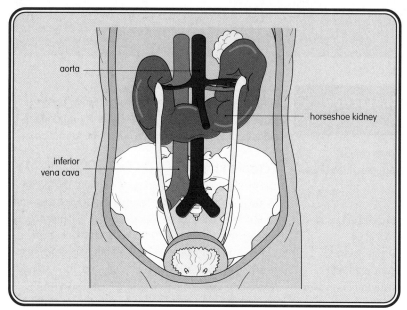

Fig. 9.2 Horseshoe kidney.

aorta

horseshoe kidney

inferior
vena cava

Describe the following congenital abnormalities of the kidney using diagrams where appropriate:
- Agenesis of the kidney.
- Hypoplasia.
- Ectopic kidney.
- Horseshoe kidney.

CYSTIC DISEASES OF THE KIDNEY

Overview

Cystic diseases of the kidney are a heterogeneous group of diseases comprising hereditary, developmental (but not hereditary), and acquired disorders. Some of these diseases can lead to chronic renal failure (CRF). Diagnosis can be made by the finding of multiple cysts on ultrasound. A single simple cyst is not an uncommon finding and should be considered normal.

Cystic renal dysplasia

This is an area of undifferentiated mesenchyme or cartilage within the parenchyma. It may occur unilaterally or bilaterally. The prognosis is better if only one kidney is affected.

Polycystic kidney disease
Adult—autosomal dominant
Incidence and presenting features

This form of polycystic kidney disease accounts for 8–10% of end-stage renal disease. Inheritance is autosomal dominant—a polycystic kidney disease (PCK) gene has been identified on chromosome 16 in the majority of cases. This disorder presents at 30–40 years of age with hypertension, urinary symptoms, or large palpable kidneys. End-stage renal failure does not normally develop until the 5th or 6th decade of life.

Pathology

Pathologically, cysts develop from dilated tubules and Bowman's capsule (Fig. 9.3) and compress the surrounding parenchyma. Sites for cyst formation are:
- Both kidneys.

- Liver (lined by biliary epithelium) in 30–40% of cases.
- Pancreas, lungs, ovaries, spleen, and other organs.

Berry aneurysms are found in 10–20% of cases. These develop as a result of congenital weakness in the artery and increased blood pressure; they may result in a subarachnoid or cerebral haemorrhage.

Macroscopically, the kidneys are large with hundreds of clear yellow fluid-filled cysts replacing the parenchyma. Haemorrhage into the cysts may occur. Microscopically, the cysts are lined by cuboidal epithelium.

Diagnosis
Diagnosis is made by:
- Ultrasound and computerized tomography (CT) in early adult life—cysts cannot reliably be found before this.
- Genetic testing in families known to carry the PCK gene.

Prognosis
Morbidity and mortality are often the result of hypertension, for example myocardial infarction and cerebrovascular disease. The condition also leads to CRF. Rarely, complications are produced by the extrarenal cysts.

Treatment
It is very important to control blood pressure. Dialysis and renal transplant are needed if CRF develops.

Child—autosomal recessive
Incidence and presenting features
This rare condition may result in stillbirth or renal failure and respiratory distress soon after birth. Some children survive for several years and develop portal hypertension and hepatic fibrosis. Inheritance is autosomal recessive and more than one gene may be involved.

Pathology
The cysts are dilated collecting ducts (Fig. 9.4); they replace the medulla and cortex and extend to the capsule. Sites involved are:
- Both kidneys.
- Liver—all children have an abnormality of the liver (cysts, bile duct cell proliferation, fibrosis interfering with liver function and leading to portal hypertension).

The macroscopic appearance is of large kidneys with a radial pattern of fusiform-like cysts.

Diagnosis, prognosis, and treatment
Diagnosis is based on the presence of a palpable mass and ultrasound findings.

The prognosis is poor and early death usually occurs due to CRF within the first few years of life unless renal replacement therapy is given.

Treatment involves managing the renal failure, hypertension, and respiratory problems.

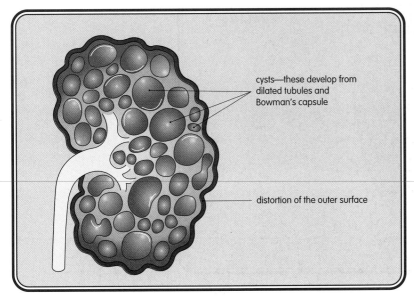

cysts—these develop from dilated tubules and Bowman's capsule

distortion of the outer surface

Fig. 9.3 Polycystic adult kidney disease.

Cystic diseases of the renal medulla
Medullary sponge kidney
Incidence and presenting features

This is uncommon. It is rarely diagnosed in children and usually presents at 30–40 years of age with symptoms of infection or stone formation.

Pathology

Dilated collecting ducts in the medulla result in cyst formation, mainly in the papillae (Fig. 9.5). Sometimes small calculi develop within the cysts. One, part of one, or both kidneys may be affected. Macroscopically some cysts are seen extending into the medulla from the involved calyces. In severe cases, the medulla looks spongy.

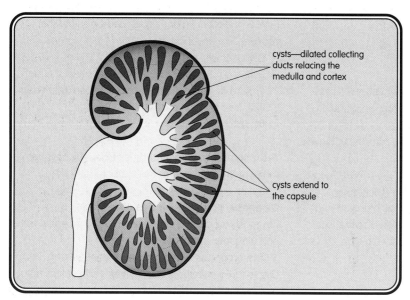

Fig. 9.4 Polycystic childhood kidney disease.

cysts—dilated collecting ducts relacing the medulla and cortex

cysts extend to the capsule

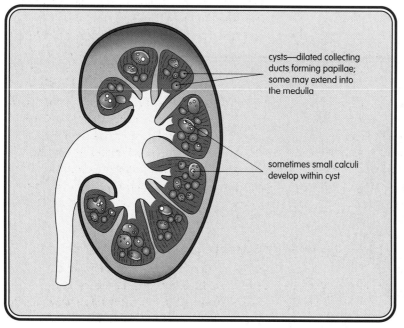

Fig. 9.5 Medullary sponge kidney.

cysts—dilated collecting ducts forming papillae; some may extend into the medulla

sometimes small calculi develop within cyst

Diagnosis, prognosis, and treatment
Diagnosis consists in intravenous urography (IVU). The prognosis is good. Renal function remains intact.

Nephronophthisis
Incidence and presenting features
This is an autosomal recessive condition that presents in early childhood. Clinical features are polydipsia, polyuria, and growth retardation. The disorder may coexist with retinal degeneration, optic atrophy, retinitis pigmentosa (giving tunnel vision—'retinal–renal syndromes'), Laurence–Moon–Biedl syndrome, or congenital hepatic fibrosis.

Pathology
Microscopically, there is interstitial inflammation and tubular atrophy. Later, medullary cysts develop.

Diagnosis, prognosis, and treatment
Diagnosis is made from the family history and renal biopsy. The disorder results in progressive renal failure, and treatment involves dialysis and renal transplantation.

Acquired cystic disease (ACD) (dialysis-associated)
ACD occurs in patients with CRF who have received dialysis for some time. The damaged kidneys contain

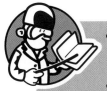

> ○ **What are the cystic diseases and how do they occur?**
> ○ **Discuss the following cystic diseases using diagrams where appropriate and note their occurrence, pathogenesis, clinical effects, and consequences:**
> —**Cystic renal dysplasia.**
> —**Polycystic kidney disease in both adult and child.**
> —**Cystic diseases of the renal medulla—medullary sponge kidney and nephronophthisis.**
> —**Acquired dialysis-associated cystic disease.**
> —**Simple cysts.**

many small cysts throughout the cortex and medulla. Obstruction of the tubules by interstitial fibrosis results in cyst formation. Oxalate crystals tend to be associated with the cysts. ACD may be associated with malignant change.

Simple cysts
The incidence of simple cysts increases with age. Their size can vary and they have a smooth lining and contain clear fluid. Renal function is not affected and pain may be felt if there is haemorrhage into the cyst. The cysts need to be differentiated from tumours— ultrasound is helpful (solid mass versus cystic mass).

DISEASES OF THE GLOMERULUS

Glomerular disease can be defined as:
- Hereditary (e.g. Alport's and Fabry's syndromes).
- Primary.
- Secondary to systemic diseases—for example diabetes mellitus, systemic lupus erythematosus (SLE), bacterial endocarditis.

Hereditary glomerular disease
Alport's syndrome
This is seen mainly in males and is X-linked. Autosomal dominant and autosomal recessive patterns of inheritance have also been described. An abnormality of basement membrane collagen IV is found in all patients and they lack the Goodpasture's antigen.

Alport's syndrome is an hereditary nephritis with haematuria, progressive renal failure and sensorineural deafness. It is associated with eye abnormalities— dislocated small lens (lenticonus), cataract, and conical cornea; platelet dysfunction; and hyperproteinaemia.

A few patients develop end-stage renal failure in childhood and adolescence. Females are usually asymptomatic carriers, but have microscopic haematuria. End-stage renal failure rarely occurs in females. The treatment consists in dialysis and/or transplantation.

Fabry's syndrome
This is an X-linked disorder, with a glycolipid metabolism defect due to the deficiency of galactosidase A. As a result, ceramide trihexosidee (a glycosphingolipid) accumulates and is deposited in the kidneys, skin, and vascular system. Death occurs in the

5th decade of life. This disorder is associated with cardiac problems such as angina and cardiac failure.

Primary

Glomerulonephritis (GN) is the term that is used to describe most glomerular diseases.

Mechanisms of glomerular injury

In-situ immune-complex deposition

Immune complexes are formed within the kidney (Fig. 9.6A). The antibodies react with intrinsic or planted antigens within the glomerulus.

Antiglomerular basement membrane (anti-GBM) disease is an example of reaction to intrinsic antigens. Antibodies are formed against an antigen in the GBM. This complex elicits the complement cascade, which then leads to severe damage to the glomerulus and rapidly progressing renal failure. The anti-GBM antibodies also attack the basement membrane of the alveoli in the lungs. The association of anti-GBM antibodies, GN, and pulmonary haemorrhage is known as Goodpasture's syndrome.

Reaction to planted antigens occurs when they are deposited within the glomerulus and are not of renal origin. They can be:

- Exogenous—for example bacteria such as group A β-haemolytic streptococci, which cause post-streptococcal GN. Other antigens include bacterial products (endostreptosin), aggregated IgG, viruses, parasites, and drugs.
- Endogenous— for example nucleic acid when antibodies react with host DNA (as seen in SLE).

Circulating immune complex nephritis

Here, immune complexes are not formed within the kidney. They are formed elsewhere and get trapped within the glomerulus after travelling to the kidney via the renal circulation (Fig. 9.6B). Once again the antigen may be:

- Exogenous—bacteria (e.g. group A streptococci such as *Treponema pallidum*), surface antigen of hepatitis B, hepatitis C virus antigen, tumour antigens, viruses.
- Endogenous—DNA in SLE.

When trapped in the glomerulus the immune complex causes an inflammatory reaction resulting in damage to the glomerulus. On immunofluorescence microscopy, granular deposits are seen to be present along the basement membrane and/or in the mesangium.

Cytotoxic antibodies

Antibodies to glomerular cell antigens cause damage without the formation and deposition of immune complexes (Fig. 9.6C). An example would be antibody fixing to mesangial cells resulting in complement-mediated mesangiolysis and mesangial cell proliferation. Experimental examples of this are known in rats, but it is not clear that this occurs in humans.

Cell-mediated immunity

Sensitized T cells from cell-mediated immune reactions can cause glomerular injury (Fig. 9.6D). This form of damage is important in progressive GN. It is thought that macrophages and T lymphocytes are present and mediate damage within the glomerulus in such cases.

Activation of alternative complement pathway

Bacterial polysaccharides, endotoxins, and IgA aggregates may activate the alternative complement pathway and give rise to components, which then deposit in the glomeruli, causing damage (Fig. 9.6E). This mechanism is seen in membranoproliferative GN.

Clinical manifestations of glomerular disease

Glomerular disease usually presents in one of the following five ways (Fig. 9.7):

- Acute nephritic syndrome.
- Nephrotic syndrome.
- Haematuria.
- Non-nephrotic levels of proteinuria.
- Chronic renal failure (CRF).

Acute nephritic syndrome

The symptoms and signs of acute nephritic syndrome are:

- Oligo/anuria.
- Hypertension.
- Fluid retention—showing as facial oedema.
- Haematuria—microscopic or macroscopic.
- Uraemia.

Several types of glomerular disease can present with this picture including:

- Post-streptococcal GN.
- Non-streptococcal GN.
- Anti-GBM disease (Goodpasture's syndrome).
- Rapidly progressive (cresenteric) GN (RPGN).
- Postinfectious RPGN.
- Focal proliferative GN.
- Mesangial IgA nephropathy (Berger's disease).

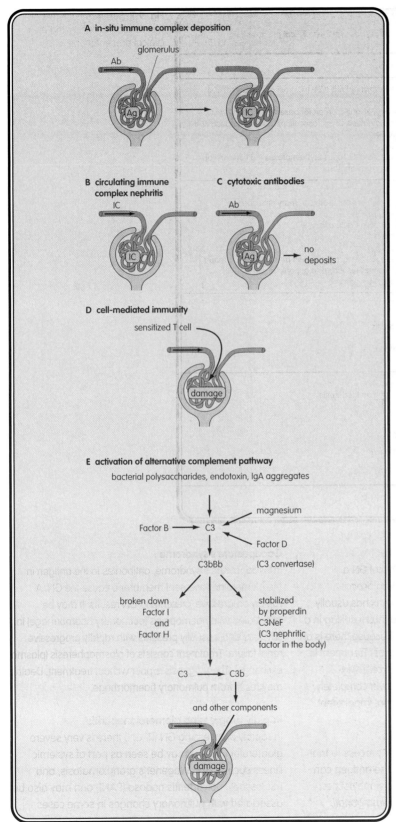

Fig. 9.6 Immune complex renal disease. (Ab, antibody; Ag, antigen; IC, immune complex.)

137

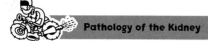

Fig. 9.7 Summary of types of glomerular diseases and their clinical presentations.

Summary of types of glomerular diseases and their clinical presentations	
Clinical presentation	**Glomerular disease**
acute nephritic syndrome	postinfection glomerulonephritis (GN) (i.e. post-streptococcal GN) non-streptococcal GN rapidly progressing GN: anti-glomerular basement membrane GN, Wegener's granulomatosis or microscopic polyarteritis nodosa (PAN) focal proliferative GN mesangial IgA GN systemic diseases: systemic lupus erythematosus (SLE), microscopic PAN, Wegener's granulomatosis
nephrotic syndrome	minimal change disease membranous glomerulonephropathy (primary or secondary) membranoproliferative GN focal segmental glomerulosclerosis shunt nephritis (rare) bacterial endocarditis (rare) systemic diseases: SLE, Henoch–Schönlein purpura (HSP), tumour, amyloid, diabetes mellitus, drugs (e.g. penicillamine, gold), congenital nephrotic syndrome
haematuria	mesangial IgA GN HSP bacterial endocarditis SLE exercise haematuria any GN
proteinuria	mesangiocapillary GN focal segmental glomerulosclerosis SLE HSP shunt nephritis polyarteritis bacterial endocarditis any GN any cause of renal scarring
chronic renal failure	any of the above diseases

Post-streptococcal glomerulonephritis

About 1–3 weeks before post-streptococcal GN a streptococcal (group A β-haemolytic streptococci) infection of either the tonsils or the pharynx has usually occurred. All the glomeruli are involved thus resulting in a diffuse proliferative GN—'proliferative' because there is an increase in the cellularity in the glomerulus. Treatment is usually conservative. The prognosis is excellent in children. Sixty per cent of adults will recover completely. The rest will develop hypertension or renal impairment.

Non-streptococcal glomerulonephritis

Non-streptococcal GN follows a similar process to that for post-streptococcal GN except that the antigen can be any organism such as bacteria (i.e. staphylococci and pneumococci), parasites (*Toxoplasma gondii, Plasmodium*), and viruses.

Goodpasture's syndrome

In Goodpasture's syndrome, antibodies to the antigen in the glomerular basement membrane cause the GN. A rapidly progressive 'cresenteric' GN results. It may be associated with haemoptysis (pulmonary haemorrhage) in smokers and it usually presents with rapidly progressive renal failure. Treatment consists of plasmapheresis (plasma exchange). The prognosis is poor without treatment. Death may result from pulmonary haemorrhage.

Rapidly progressing glomerulonephritis

In rapidly progressing GN (RPGN) there is very severe glomerular injury. It may be seen as part of systemic illness such as SLE, Wegener's granulomatosis, and microscopic polyarteritis nodosa (PAN), and may also be associated with pulmonary changes in some cases

(Wegener's granulomatosis). Histologically glomerular injury results in leakage of fibrin, which acts as a stimulus for cells (epithelial cells and macrophages) within the Bowman's capsule to proliferate and compress the glomerulus (crescent formation). As the name suggests, the disease progresses very rapidly and there is a loss of renal function within days to weeks. Treatment is plasmapheresis and immunosuppression. Hypertension, scarring of the kidney, and renal failure develop if treatment is not initiated promptly.

Postinfectious RPGN

Postinfectious RPGN is similar to RPGN but follows an infection as in post-streptococcal GN.

Focal proliferative GN

Focal proliferative GN results in inflammatory lesions in only some glomeruli. Its presentation is less acute. It may affect only the kidney (IgA nephropathy, see below) or may be part of systemic illnesses such as SLE, Henoch–Schönlein purpura (HSP), Goodpasture's syndrome, Wegener's granulomatosis, subacute bacterial endocarditis, microscopic polyarteritis. Treatment with immunosuppression is effective in some cases. The prognosis is variable.

IgA nephropathy

In mesangial IgA nephropathy, IgA and C3 are located in the mesangium of all the glomeruli associated with some mesangial proliferation. There is a urinary sediment abnormality with microscopic haematuria and proteinuria, and macroscopic haematuria in association with concurrent respiratory tract infection. IgA levels are raised with hypertension. There is some association with geographical location (more common in France, Australia, and Singapore) and HLA DR4. The treatment is non-specific. Up to 20% of patients will develop end-stage renal failure (poor prognosis group is characterized by proteinuria, increased blood pressure, and increased creatinine at presentation).

Nephrotic syndrome

In nephrotic syndrome the symptoms and signs are:
- Heavy proteinuria.
- Hypoalbuminaemia.
- Dependent generalized oedema.
- Hyperlipidaemia.

The nephrotic syndrome can be present in almost all types of GN. The most important ones are described as follows:
- Minimal change disease.
- Membranous glomerulonephropathy.
- Membranoproliferative GN.
- Focal segmental glomerulosclerosis.
- Shunt nephritis.
- Bacterial endocarditis.
- Secondary glomerular disease (e.g. diabetic nephropathy, amyloid).
- Congenital nephrotic syndrome.

Complications of nephrotic syndrome include:
- Hypercoagulable state, resulting in deep vein thrombosis (DVT), pulmonary embolus (PE) and renal vein thrombosis.
- Hyperlipidaemia, resulting in vascular disease and ischaemic heart disease.
- Immunosuppression, resulting in an increased risk of infection.

Minimal change disease

Minimal change disease is the most common cause of nephrotic syndrome in children; however, under the light microscope the kidney looks normal. Under the electron microscope there is effacement of the epithelial foot processes. The cause of minimal change disease is unknown, but potential mechanisms include a postallergic reaction, circulating immune complexes, or altered T cell immunity. Treatment consists of corticosteroid therapy. Cyclosporin or cyclophosphamide can be used in resistant cases. The prognosis is good in children and variable in adults, but usually good. Rarely (if ever) this disorder causes end-stage renal failure.

Membranous glomerulonephropathy

Membranous glomerulonephropathy is a chronic disease characterized by subepithelial deposition of immune complexes and thickening of the basement membrane. It occurs mainly in adults and in more males than females. Causes are idiopathic, primary, or secondary. Secondary causes include:
- Infections—syphilis, malaria, hepatitis B.
- Tumours—melanoma, carcinoma of the bronchus, lymphoma.
- Drugs—penicillamine, heroin, mercury, gold.
- SLE.

Drugs used to treat membranous glomerulonephropathy are corticosteroids, cyclophosphamide, cyclosporin, and chlorambucil. Thirty per cent of idiopathic cases will develop progressive CRF and require dialysis or transplantation. In membranous glomerulonephropathy due to secondary causes, the disease will usually remit with treatment of underlying disease. Complications of membranous glomerulopathy are those of any cause of the nephrotic syndrome (see above).

Membranoproliferative glomerulonephritis

In membranoproliferative GN, basement membrane thickening and mesangial proliferation occur. This is a common manifestation in children and young adults. There are three types:

- Type I—immune-complex mediated lesion (mesangiocapillary GN) with subendothelial deposits. This occurs in infections, tumours, drug reactions, genetic disorders, connective tissue disorders, and complement deficiencies.
- Type II—caused by activation of the alternative complement pathway (dense deposit disease [DDD]). This follows an infection. Immune complexes are not involved. There is an association with partial lipodystrophy.
- Type III—immune-complex deposition. The capillary walls contain many eosinophils.

Clinically, types I–III are indistinguishable. The disease progresses to end-stage renal failure and therefore has a bad prognosis. Treatment consists of dialysis and renal transplantation.

Focal segmental glomerulosclerosis

In focal segmental glomerulosclerosis there is collapse, sclerosis, and hyalinosis of focal glomerular segments. This disorder is the cause of 10% of childhood and 15% of cases of adult nephrotic syndrome. It is more common in males than females and its causes are idiopathic, altered cellular immunity, intravenous heroin use, AIDS, and reaction to chronic proteinuria; end-stage renal failure develops within 10 years. It may recur in a subsequent renal transplant. Treatment may involve steroids, cyclophosphamide, cyclosporin, dialysis, and renal transplantation.

Bacterial endocarditis

Bacterial endocarditis is discussed later.

Secondary glomerular disease

Secondary glomerular disease can occur with SLE, HSP, tumour-related immune complex disease, amyloid disease, diabetes mellitus, drug treatment (penicillamine, heroin, gold, captopril, phenytoin), infections (hepatitis B, leprosy, syphilis, malaria).

Non-specific treatment of nephrotic syndrome should include:

- The control of blood pressure
- The reduction of proteinuria—angiotensin-converting enzyme (ACE) inhibitors and non-steroidal anti-inflammatory drugs (NSAIDs) may be particularly useful.
- The control of hyperlipidaemia.
- Anticoagulation if hypercoagulable.

Haematuria

Haematuria due to glomerular disease is often painless; it is not associated with any other urinary symptoms. Possible glomerular diseases include:

- Mesangial IgA nephropathy.
- Bacterial endocarditis.
- SLE.
- HSP.
- Polyarteritis.
- Wegener's granulomatosis.
- Any GN.

Heavy exercise may result in haemoglobinuria (not haematuria).

Non-nephrotic levels of proteinuria

This is characterized by proteinuria (usually up to 3 g protein daily in the urine) with no other symptoms. Possible causes are:

- Mesangiocapillary GN.
- Focal segmental glomerulosclerosis.
- SLE.
- IgA.
- Severe or longstanding hypertension.
- HSP.
- Shunt nephritis.
- Polyarteritis.
- Wegener's granulomatosis.
- Bacterial endocarditis.
- Any GN.
- Any disease causing renal scarring including chronic pyelonephritis.

Chronic renal failure

Many of the diseases mentioned above can cause chronic renal failure (CRF). This is often asymptomatic in the early stages. When advanced, it presents with:

- Uraemia.
- Hypertension.
- Salt and water retention causing oedema.
- Anaemia.
- Nausea, vomiting, diarrhoea.
- Gastrointestinal bleeding.
- Itching.
- Polyuria and nocturia.
- Lethargy.
- Paraesthesiae (due to polyneuropathy).
- Mental slowing and clouding of consciousness.

In extreme cases, oliguria results. The only treatment is dialysis until renal transplantation is possible. In CRF the kidney contracts with thinning of the cortex. Most of the glomeruli consist of hyaline balls and there is almost complete tubular atrophy.

- How is glomerular disease classified?
- Discuss the main developmental mechanisms of glomerular disease.
- Discuss the five main clinical syndromes associated with the clinical manifestations of glomerular disease giving examples of and briefly explaining the diseases that present in this way.

GLOMERULAR LESIONS IN SYSTEMIC DISEASE

Systemic disorders can cause glomerular disease. They are usually:

- Immune-complex mediated (e.g. SLE, HSP, bacterial endocarditis).
- Vascular (e.g. PAN, Wegener's granulomatosis).
- Metabolic (e.g. diabetes mellitus, amyloidosis).

Systemic lupus erythematosus (SLE)

SLE is a condition that affects many systems and organs in the body, for example the joints, skin, heart, lungs, serosal membranes, and the kidneys (70% of cases). The glomerular diseases seen are:

- Diffuse proliferative GN.
- Focal proliferative GN.
- Membranous glomerulopathy.

Henoch–Schönhein purpura (HSP)

HSP is most common in children. It is a systemic vasculitis affecting many parts of the body including:

- Skin—a purpuric rash is seen over on the extensor side of the legs and arms and buttocks.
- Joints—resulting in pain.
- Intestine—resulting in abdominal pain, vomiting, bleeding.
- Kidney—resulting in GN (in about one-third of patients) indistinguishable from IgA nephropathy.

HSP seems to be associated with a previous upper respiratory tract infection. It has an excellent prognosis in children.

Bacterial endocarditis

It is thought that the glomerular disease in bacterial endocarditis is caused by immune complex deposition. The main histological abnormalities are focal, segmental, and diffuse proliferative GN. It is also possible that emboli break away from the heart valves and causes kidney infarcts.

Diabetic glomerulosclerosis

Diabetes mellitus affects several systems and organs in the body including the eyes, vascular system, and kidneys. This is mainly because it damages all the large and small vessels in the body. End-stage renal failure occurs in 30% of cases of insulin-dependent type I diabetes mellitus. Diabetic nephropathy presents with the development of microalbunuria. This progresses through non-nephrotic range and then nephrotic range proteinuria, following which there is a progressive fall in GFR leading to CRF. It is also associated with diabetic complications elsewhere (e.g. retinopathy). Increased blood pressure is a common feature. The arteries may also be affected (especially in type II) and severe atheroma in the renal artery will cause renal ischaemic lesions and hypertension. Papillary necrosis is a recognized complication, especially in the presence of infection. Histological features can include:

- Thickening of the basement membrane.
- Increase in the matrix of the mesangium.
- A diffuse or nodular pattern of glomerulosclerosis (also known as Kimmelstiel–Wilson syndrome).
- Arterial hyalinosis of both the afferent and efferent arterioles.

Amyloidosis

This disorder involves the kidneys in 80–90% of patients. There are amyloid deposits in the glomeruli, usually within the mesangium and subendothelium and sometimes in the subepithelial space. Some deposits may also be found in the walls of the blood vessels and in the interstitium. The commonest presentation is heavy proteinuria or the nephrotic syndrome. CRF usually results when the main histological lesions are those of glomerulosclerosis. Death results from uraemia unless renal replacement treatment is given.

Microscopic polyarteritis nodosa (PAN)

This disorder involves the small arteries in the body. Initially there is a focal, segmental, or necrotizing GN followed by RPGN (with extensive necrosis, fibrin deposition and epithelial crescents). Microscopic PAN is associated with circulating antineutrophil cytoplasmic antibodies (ANCA). These characteristically recognize a perinuclear antigen in fixed neutrophils (pANCA).

Wegener's granulomatosis

This is a rare disease in which a necrotizing vasculitis affects the nose, upper respiratory tract, and kidneys. The glomerular disease is similar to that for microscopic PAN. It is associated with ANCA, which characteristically recognizes a cytoplasmic antigen in fixed neutrophils (cANCA).

Discuss how the following systemic diseases affect the kidney:
- SLE.
- HSP.
- Bacterial endocarditis.
- Diabetic glomerulosclerosis.
- Amyloidosis.
- PAN.
- Wegener's granulomatosis.

Hereditary nephritis

This disorder is associated with a familial inheritance of glomerular injury (e.g. Alport's syndrome, see p. 135).

DISEASES OF THE TUBULES AND INTERSTITIUM

Acute tubular necrosis (ATN)

ATN is the result of acute tubular cell damage. It may be oliguric (up to 400 mL/day urine passed) or non-oliguric. There is a risk of hyperkalaemia due to K^+ retention and this can trigger cardiac arrhythmias, which can be life-threatening. Uraemia develops because of a marked decrease in GFR—this may be due to haemodynamic changes and intratubular obstruction. Recovery is accompanied by a diuretic phase that occurs because of failure to concentrate urine and this can cause hypokalaemia.

ATN is a cause of acute renal failure (ARF). It carries a 50% mortality, but potentially a full recovery is possible with adequate fluid and electrolyte therapy and dialysis if necessary. The commonest causes of ATN are:

- Severe acute ischaemia.
- Toxins.

Careful management and resuscitation of critically ill patients can decrease the incidence of ATN.

Ischaemic ATN

This is caused by shock following trauma, infections, burns, crush injury, or haemorrhage (e.g. postpartum haemorrhage, gastrointestinal bleeding, or stabbing). The rapid fall in blood pressure that occurs leads to hypotension, which causes hypoperfusion of the peritubular capillaries and results in tubular necrosis along the entire length of the nephron. The kidneys appear pale and swollen. On histology there is an infiltration of inflammatory cells and the tubular cells appear flattened and vacuolated. There is interstitial oedema. Casts of cellular debris and protein (Tamm-Horsfall protein) are found in the distal tubule and the collecting ducts. Myoglobin is found in the casts in crush injuries. NSAIDs may predispose patients to ATN in the face of other renal insults by preventing the synthesis of vasodilator prostaglandins which would normally protect the kidney from ischaemic injury.

Toxic ATN

This disorder is caused by substances that have specific nephrotoxic activity and that damage the epithelial cells. Such substances include:

- Organic solvents—carbon tetrachloride (CCl_4) in dry-cleaning fluid.
- Heavy metals (gold, mercury, lead, and arsenic).
- Antibiotics (gentamicin).
- Pesticides.

These substances cause the cells to come away from the basement membrane and consequently collect in and obstruct the tubular lumen. The effect is limited since there is regeneration of the epithelial cells in 10–20 days, which permits clinical recovery and is confirmed by the presence of mitotic figures on biopsy. Damage by nephrotoxic substances is limited to the proximal tubules. The kidneys appear swollen and red.

Tubulointerstitial nephritis

Urinary tract infection (UTI)

Incidence and risk factors

UTIs are very common in the general population. They can involve the bladder (cystitis) or the kidneys (pyelonephritis) or both. At birth there is a greater incidence in boys due to congenital abnormalities; this is reversed at pre-school age with the highest incidence then occurring in girls and women (sex ratio 20:1) up to the age of 45–50 years when prostatic disease in men results in an increased incidence of UTI in men. Women are particularly at risk of lower urinary tract infections because they have a short urethra. Risk factors for UTIs include:

- Long-term catheterization.
- Diabetes mellitus.
- Lower urinary tract obstruction (congenital abnormalities or calculi).
- Pregnancy.
- Tumours.
- Immunosuppression.

Presentation

UTIs present silently (asymptomatic bacteriuria) or with dysuria (pain on passing urine), frequency, and urgency of micturition. Involvement of the kidneys causes loin pain and fever.

Diagnosis

A diagnosis of UTI requires over 10^5 CFU/mL from a mid-stream urine specimen on culture. In the majority of UTIs the infecting organism comes from the patient's own faecal flora (Fig. 9.8).

Pyelonephritis

This is a bacterial infection of the kidney and results in inflammation and damage to the renal calyces, parenchyma, and pelvis. It may be acute or chronic.

Acute pyelonephritis

This occurs because of infection in the kidney and is spread via two routes:

- Retrograde ureteric spread—the organism can only gain access to the kidney from the lower urinary tract if there is an incompetent vesico-ureteric valve; this permits vesico-ureteric reflux (VUR) and results in ascending transmission of infection.
- Haematogenous spread—this method occurs in patients with septicaemia or infective endocarditis. The pathogens include fungi, bacteria (staphylococci and *Escherichia coli*) and viruses. The kidney is often affected in septicaemic diseases because of its large blood supply.

The predisposing factors of acute pyelonephritis are:

- Urinary tract obstruction (congenital and acquired).
- VUR.
- Instrumentation of the urinary tract.

Incidence of community- and hospital-acquired UTIs caused by bacteria		
Organism	**Community (%)**	**Hospital (%)**
Escherichia coli	80–90	45–55
Proteus	5–10	10–12
Klebsiella	1–2	15–20
Enterobacter	–	2–5
Pseudomonas	–	10–15
Acinetobacter	–	<1
coagulase-negative *Staphylococcus*	1–2	1–2
Staphylococcus aureus	–	<1
Enterococcus	<1	10–12

Fig. 9.8 Incidence of community- and hospital-acquired urinary tract infections (UTIs) caused by bacteria.

- Sexual intercourse.
- Diabetes.
- Immunosuppression (HIV, lymphoma, and transplants).

Patients present with general malaise, fever, loin pain, tenderness, and often rigors. There may or may not be symptoms of infection in the lower urinary tract. Infection spreads into the renal pelvis and papillae and causes abscess formation throughout the cortex and medulla.

With retrograde ureteric spread the kidney characteristically contains areas of wedge-shaped suppuration especially at the upper and lower poles. In septicaemia there is haematogenous seeding within the kidney and minute abscesses are distributed randomly in the cortex. On histology there is:
- Polymorphic infiltration of the tubules.
- Interstitial oedema.
- Inflammation.
Fibrosis occurs on healing.

Uncomplicated cases resolve in a few days with antibiotic treatment. The important complications of acute pyelonephritis are:
- Renal papillary necrosis.
- Perinephric abscesses.
- Pyonephrosis.

Chronic pyelonephritis

This is defined as long-standing parenchymal scarring and is the end-result of various pathological processes. It is often associated with VUR, which occurs as a result of congenital abnormalities early in life or acquired obstruction in adults. There are two main pathological processes that result in chronic pyelonephritis:
- Obstructive—any chronic obstruction (stones, tumours, or congenital abnormalities) will predispose the kidney to infection and the chronic pyelonephritis develops due to recurrent infection.
- Reflux neuropathy—this is the most common cause of chronic pyelonephritis. The organisms enter the ascending portion of the ureter with refluxed urine as the valvular orifice is maintained open on contraction of the bladder during micturition. This is due to the abnormal angle at which the terminal ureter enters the bladder wall (Fig. 9.9).

The disease process usually begins in childhood and has a silent, insidious onset. Reflux of urine into the renal pelvis occurs during micturition and this increases the pressure in the major calyces. The high intrapelvic pressure facilitates reflux into the collecting ducts with intraparenchymal reflux further distorting the internal structure. This is most predominant at the poles of the kidney and results in deep irregular scars on the cortical

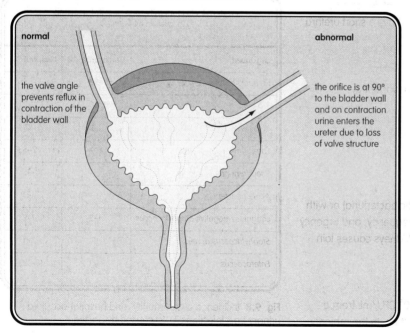

Fig. 9.9 Normal and refluxing (abnormal) junction.

normal

the valve angle prevents reflux in contraction of the bladder wall

abnormal

the orifice is at 90° to the bladder wall and on contraction urine enters the ureter due to loss of valve structure

surface. The tubulointerstitial inflammation heals with the formation of corticomedullary scars that overlie the deformed and dilated calyces, which are characteristic of chronic pyelonephritis (Fig. 9.10).

On histology there is fibrosis of the interstitium and there are dilated tubules containing eosinophilic casts. Approximately 10–20% of patients with CRF requiring renal replacement therapy have chronic pyelonephritis.

Diagnosis is made by IVP (see Chapter 8), which shows distortion of the calyceal system and contraction of the kidney due to cortical scarring. Generally, radiographs are avoided in children. Ultrasonography is also used to diagnose chronic pyelonephritis, but the isotope renogram is the more sensitive technique.

Any UTI in children and adult males should be investigated to exclude an underlying renal tract abnormality. UTI is common in adult females but, if recurrent, further investigation is indicated. UTI rarely progresses to renal damage in adults if the renal tract is normal. High fluid intake, regular bladder drainage and prophylactic antibiotics are the mainstay of treatment.

Toxin-induced interstitial nephritis

Heavy metals (mercury, gold, lead) and drugs (ampicillin, rifampicin, NSAIDs) can cause a T cell-mediated inflammatory reaction in the interstitium. The reaction usually occurs within 2–40 days after ingestion of the toxin and withdrawal of the drug promotes

recovery within the renal tissue. The signs include fever, skin rash, haematuria, mild proteinuria, and ARF.

On histology there is interstitial oedema and tubular degeneration; eosinophils are the predominant cell type.

In chronic analgesic abuse the patient usually consumes a mixture of phenacetin-containing drugs and aspirin, which has an ischaemic effect on the kidney by inhibiting the synthesis of prostaglandins. This causes papillary necrosis and then a secondary tubulonephritis (analgesic nephropathy). There is an increased risk of developing transitional cell carcinomas with chronic analgesic abuse.

Urate nephropathy

Urate crystals can be deposited in the distal nephron in the medulla of the kidney if there are raised blood levels of urate concentration. The urate crystals that precipitate in the acidic environment of the distal nephron cause obstruction and dilatation of the tubules and eventually become surrounded by fibrosis. An increase in urate concentration can be due to a rapid turnover of cells (e.g. in psoriasis or malignancy) or due to decreased uric acid clearance (e.g. in CRF). In patients with haematological or lymphatic malignancy who are receiving chemotherapy, the excessive cell breakdown and release of nucleic acids can result in acute urate nephropathy and ARF ('tumour lysis syndrome'). CRF can also occur in patients with gout in which there is a long-

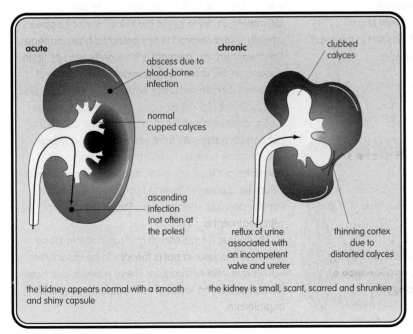

Fig. 9.10 Differences between acute and chronic pyelonephritis.

acute

- abscess due to blood-borne infection
- normal cupped calyces
- ascending infection (not often at the poles)

the kidney appears normal with a smooth and shiny capsule

chronic

- clubbed calyces
- reflux of urine associated with an incompetent valve and ureter
- thinning cortex due to distorted calyces

the kidney is small, scant, scarred and shrunken

term deposition of urate in the kidney due to the constant high levels of uric acid in the blood.

Hypercalcaemia

A constant high level of Ca^{2+} in the blood causes Ca^{2+} deposition in the kidneys. The hypercalcaemia may be due to:

- Primary hyperparathyroidism.
- Multiple myeloma.
- Increased vitamin D activity.
- Bone metastases.

Renal insufficiency occurs in these patients because of stones (nephrolithiasis) or focal calcification due to Ca^{2+} deposition in the kidney (nephrocalcinosis).

In nephrocalcinosis the Ca^{2+} accumulates in the tubular cells and then on the basement membrane resulting in interstitial fibrosis and inflammation. Hypercalcaemia also causes a renal concentrating defect which leads to polyuria, nocturia, and dehydration.

Multiple myeloma

Approximately 50% of patients with myeloproliferative disorders develop renal insufficiency, which can cause ARF or CRF. This occurs in one of the following ways:

- Bence Jones proteins (light chains) are lost in the urine and these are toxic to the tubular epithelial cells. They combine with Tamm–Horsfall protein to form inflammatory and obstructive casts in the tubules that erode into the interstitium.
- Amyloid lambda (λ) or kappa (κ) light chain fragments (paraproteins) are deposited in the renal blood vessels, glomeruli, and tubules.
- Urate deposition (see above).
- Hypercalcaemia (see above).

- **What are the causes of ATN?**
- **Discuss the incidence, presentation, and diagnosis of UTIs.**
- **For acute and chronic pyelonephritis discuss the aetiology, prediposing factors, appearance of the kidney, and histology.**

DISEASES OF THE RENAL BLOOD VESSELS

Benign nephrosclerosis

This is the term given to the changes in renal vasculature induced by essential (benign) hypertension. The changes consist of hyaline arteriolosclerosis, which is characterized by thickening (due to hyperplasia of smooth muscle) and hyalinization (protein deposition) of the arteriolar wall. This causes narrowing of the lumen of the interlobular arteries. The larger branches of the arteries are not functionally compromised. The changes are more severe in patients with diabetes and other systemic diseases with manifestations in the renal vessels. Because of the vascular wall lesions there is a compromised blood supply to the kidney, which leads to ischaemic atrophy of the nephrons. This accounts for the small, contracted, and granular appearance of the kidneys seen in advanced cases of untreated essential hypertension. Proteinuria is a common complication as a result of glomerular damage. Renal function rarely deteriorates if the blood pressure is controlled.

Malignant nephrosclerosis

This is associated with accelelerated hypertension. It occurs in 1–5% of patients with essential hypertension. There is a sudden accelerated rise in blood pressure with an increase in diastolic pressure to over 130 mmHg. In acute cases the kidney surface appears smooth and is covered in tiny petechial haemorrhages. Renal vascular involvement is frequently seen as fibrin deposits in the vessel wall associated with areas of necrosis (fibrinoid necrosis), especially in the distal part of the interlobular arteries and the afferent arteroles.

An effect on renal function is inevitable due to the ischaemia that results from severe arterial damage. Patients may have massive proteinuria and haematuria, and if untreated frequently develop renal failure (in contrast to benign hypertension). Papilloedema is often present. The 5-year survival rate with treatment is 50%.

The trigger for the abrupt and rapid rise in blood pressure is unknown but is thought to be associated with endothelial dysfunction. These patients also have increased plasma levels of renin, aldosterone, and angiotensin.

Renal artery stenosis

In 2–5% of patients with hypertension, the hypertension is secondary to renal artery stenosis (RAS) in one or both renal arteries. The stenoses are due to fibromuscular dysplasia or atheromatous plaques (70%) within the renal artery wall (Fig. 9.11). The renal hypoperfusion is interpreted by the affected kidney as a fall in body fluid volume and results in excessive renin secretion. There is also some renal ischaemia.

Treatment to dilate the stenosis (angioplasty) or corrective surgery may aid blood pressure control and preserve renal function. If the blood pressure is left uncontrolled the contralateral kidney may become damaged by hypertension.

Thrombotic microangiopathies

This is a group of diseases that are all characterized by necrosis and thickening of the renal vessel walls and thrombosis in the interlobular arterioles, afferent arterioles, and glomeruli. The clinical manifestations include ARF, thrombocytopenia, and a microangiopathic haemolytic anaemia. The diseases include:

- Haemolytic uraemic syndrome (HUS).
- Thrombotic thrombocytopaenic purpura (TTP).
- Disseminated intravascular coagulation (DIC).

Haemolytic uraemic syndrome (HUS)

There are three types of HUS:

- Childhood.
- Adult.
- Secondary.

The features of all three subtypes are a triad of:

- Microangiopathic haemolytic anaemia.
- Thrombocytopenia.
- Acute nephropathy.

As erythrocytes pass through fibrin strands that are deposited in arterioles, they are destroyed, giving rise to characteristic bur-shaped and helmet-shaped cell.

Childhood (classic) HUS

Classic HUS is the most common renal cause of ARF in childhood. There is an initial prodromal flu-like illness or gastrointestinal infection causing bloody diarrhoea (this is also called diarrhoea-associated HUS) in which it is thought that there is a activation of a neutrophil-mediated reaction, which damages the vascular endothelium.

Approximately 70–80% of the patients have an infection of the verocytotoxin-producing *E. coli* (subtype O157).

The prodromal illness is followed by the sudden onset of oliguria and haematuria, occasionally with melaena, and rarely with haematemesis. Other organs including the brain and heart may also be involved, and such involvement is associated with a worse prognosis and resistance to treatment. The platelet count is reduced but clotting is normal.

Treatment includes early supportive therapy with dialysis. The prognosis is much better in children than in adults. Fresh frozen plasma may be helpful. About 50% of patients develop hypertension and a few go on to develop CRF.

Adult HUS

This is similar to the syndrome that occurs in childen. It occurs in association with:

- Infection—typhoid fever, *E. coli* infection and shigellosis.
- Pregnancy—pre-eclampsia and postpartum renal failure.
- Oestrogen therapy—oral contraceptive pill.

Adult HUS is much more serious than HUS in children and more frequently fatal.

Secondary HUS

This disorder occurs as a complication of conditions associated with other vascular renal disease such as

Contrasting clinical findings of fibromuscular dysplasia and atheromatous RAS		
	Fibromuscular dysplasia	**Atheromatous RAS**
age (years)	<40	>55
sex prevalence	F > M	M > F
bruit heard	80%	40%
vascular disease elsewhere	rare	common
renal failure	rare	well recognized
patient prognosis	good	poor

Fig. 9.11 Contrast between fibromuscular dysplasia and atheromatous renal artery stenosis (RAS).

SLE, malignant hypertension, scleroderma, and transplant rejection. It can also occur on administration of cyclosporin A.

Thrombotic thrombocytopaenic purpura

This is a rare and idiopathic condition. The features are fever, neurological signs (CNS involvement), haemolytic anaemia, and thrombocytopaenia. It is similar to HUS except that there is renal involvement in only 50% of cases, which presents as:

- Proteinuria.
- Haematuria.
- Renal insufficiency.

The majority of cases have a dominant CNS component. The disorder is more common in women, especially in those under 40 years of age.

On histology thrombi consisting of fibrin and platelets are found in the terminal interlobular arteries, the afferent arterioles, and glomerular capillaries.

Mortality is high since there is no effective treatment at present. Fresh frozen plasma and immunosupressive treatments have been used.

Disseminated intravascular coagulation

This is a systemic condition that occurs when the coagulation cascade is activated by a stimulus that results in fibrin–platelet thrombi in blood vessels. This stimulates the process of fibrinolysis and as the two processes continue in parallel the result is a depletion of platelets, clotting factors, and excessive bleeding. Fibrin thrombi can become lodged in the glomerular capillaries, obstructing the lumen and causing severe renal damage.

The causes of DIC include Gram-negative septicaemia, amniotic fluid embolism, dead fetus, malignant disease of the lung, pancreas, and prostate, shock, and dialysis.

Renal infarction
Embolic infarction

The embolus can come from:

- Thrombotic material from the left side of the heart.
- Atheromatous material from plaques.
- Bacterial vegetations from infective endocarditis.

The emboli lodge in the small renal vessels and cause narrowing of the arterioles and focal areas of ischaemic

injury. Presentation can be silent or with haematuria and loin tenderness. The areas of infarction appear pale and are characteristically wedge shaped.

Diffuse cortical necrosis

Diffuse cortical necrosis causes ARF and presents with anuria. This is a rare condition that occurs as a complication of:

- Severe haemorrhage.
- Sepsis.

As a result of profound hypotension in these disorders there is compensatory vasoconstriction that can cause infarction. This can be avoided by prompt resuscitation of the shocked patient. Once the disease is established, no agent has been shown to improve outcome. Prognosis is much better for focal infarction than for generalized cortical infarction. The surface of the kidney appears patchy with irregular yellow areas on a background of congestion and haemorrhage which is limited to the cortex. Infarcts may calcify with time.

- Outline the changes seen in the renal vasculature in hypertension.
- Outline the differences between the two types of renal artery stenosis.
- List the characteristic features of HUS and discuss the three types.

NEOPLASTIC DISEASE OF THE KIDNEY

Benign tumours of the kidney
Renal fibroma

Renal fibroma is the commonest benign renal tumour. It is a small (less than 1 cm diameter) firm, well demarcated, white nodule. The nodule is made up of fibroblast-like cells and collagen. It is often an incidental finding in the renal medulla and has no clinical significance.

Cortical adenoma

This is a small (less than 3 cm diameter) discrete, yellowish-grey nodule. It is an incidental finding in 20–25% of autopsies. On histology it is found to be composed of large vacuolated clear cells with small nuclei. (This is identical to the histological appearance of a renal cell carcinoma.) The diagnosis is usually made from the size of the tumour:

- Less than 30 mm diameter—benign.
- Over 30 mm diameter—malignant.

Cortical adenomas have a low malignant potential.

Angiomyolipoma

This is also called a hamartomatous malformation. The tumour is made up of blood vessels, muscle, and mature fat. Angiomyolipomas are associated with tuberous sclerosis, which is an inherited disease that involves the central nervous system, skin, and other viscera.

Oncocytoma

This is an epithelial cell tumour. It can grow to a diameter of 12 cm, but never metastasizes. On histology the cytoplasm is seen to have a granular appearance due to the vast number of mitochondria in the tumour cells.

Malignant tumours of the kidney
Renal cell carcinoma (RCC)
Incidence and risk factors

Approximately 90% of renal malignant tumours in adults are RCCs (adenocarcinomas that arise from the tubular epithelium). RCC is very rare in children and has a peak incidence in 60–70 year olds. The male to female ratio is 3:1. It has great geographical variance with the highest incidence in Scandinavia and the lowest in South America and Africa. The predisposing factors are:

- Acquired cystic disease in patients who require renal replacement therapy carries a 50-fold increased risk of RCC, which tends to occur at a much earlier age than in the normal population.
- Von Hippel–Lindau disease, which is a rare inherited disease due to a deletion in the 3p gene on chromosome 25. Tenty per cent of these patients develop RCC.

There is an increased incidence of RCC among smokers.

Presentation

The tumour presents as haematuria in 90% of cases. Non-specific symptoms include fatigue, weight loss, and fever. There may be a mass in the loin. These are all late manifestations, presenting at an advanced stage of tumour progression and this explains the poor prognosis of RCC. Approximately 10% of RCCs are clinically silent and present as metastatic disease (occult primary).

A small number of RCCs can secrete hormone-like substances such as:

- Parathyroid hormone (PTH), resulting in hypercalcaemia.
- Adrenocorticotrophic hormone (ACTH), resulting in a Cushing's-like syndrome.
- Erythropoietin, resulting in polycythaemia.
- Renin, resulting in hypertension.

As a result of these hormone-producing tumours, RCC commonly presents with paraneoplastic syndromes.

Diagnosis

Diagnosis is made by IVU (revealing a space-occupying lesion in the kidney that distorts the outline), ultrasonography, and CT (see Chapter 8).

Pathology

RCC consists of a yellow–brown well-demarcated mass in the renal cortex with a diameter of 3–15 cm. Within this area there are patches of haemorrhage, necrosis, and cyst formation. The tumours are most common at the upper pole of the kidney. The renal capsule is often intact, although it can be breached and the tumour will extend into the perinephric fat. Spread in to the renal vein is often visible and rarely this extends into the inferior vena cava.

On histology the tumour is seen to contain cells with clear cytoplasm that range from well differentiated to anaplastic.

Spread takes place by direct invasion of local tissues, via the lymph to lumbar nodes (one-third of cases), and via the blood (venous). Metastases are found in the lung, liver, bone, opposite kidney, and adrenals. RCC often metastasizes before local symptoms occur.

Prognosis

The prognosis of RCC is unpredictable and is generally determined by the degree of the spread; staging of RCC is performed by assessing local, nodal, and metastatic

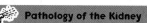
spread (TNM classification).

- T_1—confined to the kidney.
- T_2—enlarging tumour with distortion of the kidney with renal capsule intact.
- T_3—spread through the renal capsule into the perinephric fat with invasion into the renal vein.
- T_4—invasion into adjacent organs or the abdominal wall.
- N^+—lymph node involvement.
- M^+—metastatic spread.

Treatment

The treatment of choice for RCC if there are no distant metastases is a radical nephrectomy with removal of the associated adrenal gland, perinephric fat, upper ureter, and the para-aortic lymph nodes. There is little effective treatment available for metastatic disease. The average 5-year survival rate is 45% and if there is no metastatic disease on presentation it increases to 70%.

Wilms' tumour (nephroblastoma)

Incidence and presentation

Nephroblastoma is the commonest malignant tumour in children. The peak incidence is in 1–4 year olds. There is no sex preference. It is an embryonic tumour derived from the primitive metanephros. It presents with an abdominal mass and occasionally haematuria, abdominal pain, and hypertension.

Pathology

The tumours are large solid masses of firm white tissue with areas of necrosis and haemorrhage. They often breach the renal capsule and grow into the perinephric fat. On histology they are seen to be composed of characteristic spindle cells or primitive blastema cells with epithelial and mesenchymal tissues, cartilage, bone, and muscle. They are aggressive tumours and often there is metastatic disease of the lung on presentation.

Treatment and prognosis

Treatment involves surgical resection of the tumour with a combination of radiotherapy and chemotherapy. The long-term survival rate is over 80%.

The prognosis depends upon the extent of the tumour and distant spread at the time of diagnosis.

Urothelial carcinoma of the renal pelvis

This is a transitional cell tumour arising from the renal pelvis. Aetiological factors include:

- Analgesic abuse.
- Exposure to aniline dyes used in the industrial manufacture of dyes, rubber, and plastics.

Urothelial carcinoma of the renal pelvis presents early with haematuria or as an obstructive lesion because it projects directly into the pelvicalyceal cavity.

The tumours range from well-differentiated tumours to diffuse, invasive, and anaplastic carcinomas. The poorly differentiated tumours are associated with a poor prognosis and often invade the wall of the renal pelvis and involve the renal vein. Multiple tumours are also often found in the ureters and bladder. Fragments of papillary tumour fronds and atypical tumour cells can be detected in the urine and this makes cytological diagnosis possible.

- ○ **Name the four types of benign renal tumour.**
- ○ **Discuss renal cell carcinoma noting its incidence, age group affected, predisposing factors, presentation, and morphology.**
- ○ **What is a Wilms' tumour? What age group does it affect?**

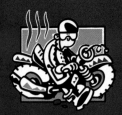

10. Pathology of the Urinary Tract

CONGENITAL ABNORMALITIES OF THE URINARY TRACT

Abnormalities associated with development of the kidneys are discussed in Chapter 1.

Ureteric abnormalities
These occur in 2–5% of the population and usually have little clinical relevance. Infrequently they are associated with an obstruction of urine flow (see Chapter 10).

Double and bifid ureters
The ureters along with the calyces and collecting ducts are formed from an outgrowth of the mesonephric (wolffian) duct called the ureteric bud. Early splitting of the ureteric bud or the development of two buds results in the development of double (bifid) ureters (Fig. 10.1). The duplication may be partial or complete. It is often associated with double renal pelvises with their own renal parenchyma or more frequently with a number of lobes in common. Renal function is rarely compromised. Reflux may occur up one moiety. There is a strong predisposition to infection.

Ureteropelvic junction obstruction
This disorder presents in infants, especially in males, and is more common in the left ureter. It is bilateral in 20% of cases and is thought to occur as a result of abnormal smooth muscle organization at the ureteropelvic junction. In some cases it may be accompanied by renal agenesis of the opposite kidney. The reason for this is unknown. As a result of the back pressure from the obstruction, dilatation of the pelvicalyceal system (Fig. 10.2) may occur, and if the pressure is transmitted up to the kidneys there is atrophy of the renal tissue.

Diverticula
Diverticula are outpouchings of the ureteral wall and are very common. The majority are congenital and create sites for stasis of urine. This predisposes the urine to infection since one of the main barriers to infection in the urinary tract is the continuous flushing through of urine. Acquired diverticula may appear as a result of increased pressure in the ureters.

Hydroureter and megaloureter
Congenital hydroureters occur as a result of a neuromuscular defects in the wall of the ureter and are

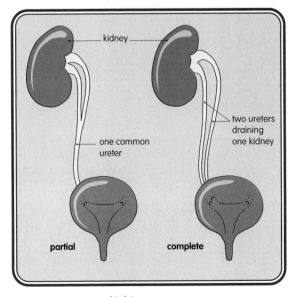

Fig. 10.1 Two types of bifid ureter.

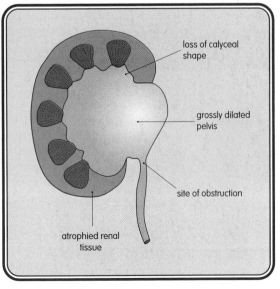

Fig. 10.2 Pelvicalyceal dilatation.

often associated with other congenital malformations in the genitourinary tract. There is dilatation, elongation, and frequently tortuosity of the ureters. Megaloureter is the name given to massive enlargement of the ureter. Acquired hydroureters occur in adults during pregnancy and lower urinary tract obstruction.

Bladder abnormalities
Diverticula
These are sac-like outpouchings of the bladder wall. They can be either congenital or acquired as a result of chronic urethral obstruction:

- The congenital diverticula develop in localized areas of defective muscle within the wall or are due to urinary tract obstruction in fetal development. They are usually solitary lesions.
- Acquired diverticula are multiple and most commonly develop much later in life in association with prostatic hypertrophy. They are clinically significant since they act as sites of urinary stasis and predispose to bladder infection and the development of vesico-ureteric reflux.

Exstrophy
Exstrophy of the bladder is a serious condition affecting the anterior wall of the bladder and anterior abdominal wall. As a result of failure in development of the anterior wall of the bladder, the posterior wall is directly exposed to the external environment (the bladder has the appearance of being turned inside out) and there is squamous metaplasia of the mucosa. The mucosa is at high risk of infection. This disorder is often associated with urethral and symphysis pubis defects. In the male there is epispadias and in females a split clitoris. There is an increased risk of adenocarcinomas of the bladder associated with extrusion of the bladder. Surgical correction allows long-term survival of these infants.

Urethral abnormalities
Hypospadias
Approximately 3–4 in every 1000 male infants are affected to a varying degree. The urethra opens on the ventral surface of the penis, usually adjacent to the glans penis, but may open on the penile shaft or perineum. There is a ventral curvature to the penile shaft. Surgical correction is carried out before two years of age to allow micturation while standing.

Epispadias
The urethra opens on the dorsal surface of the penis. As with hypospadias surgical correction is carried out before two years of age to allow micturation while standing.

Urethral valves
Obstruction to urine flow can occur at the level of the posterior urethra in a boy due to the presence of mucosal folds or a membrane (posterior urethral valve). A male fetus with a posterior urethral valve may have poor renal growth, progressive bilateral hydronephrosis, and oligohydramnios (decreased volume of amniotic fluid) as a result of severe obstruction to urinary flow.

Intrauterine intervention has no proven benefit and an early delivery is only performed if there are signs of rapidly progressing renal damage. Postnatal management includes:

- Prophylactic antibiotic from birth to prevent urinary tract infection (UTI).
- Ultrasound scans at birth and a few weeks later to assess the effect of the obstruction.

Surgical treatment is required in all cases. Further investigations of any male child born with bilateral hydronephrosis are required to exclude a posterior urethral valve.

Describe the following congenital abnormalities of the urinary tract using diagrams where appropriate:
- **Double and bifid ureters.**
- **Ureteropelvic junction obstruction.**
- **Bladder and ureteric diverticula.**
- **Hydroureter.**
- **Bladder exstrophy.**
- **Hypospadias and epispadias.**
- **Urethral valves.**

URINARY TRACT OBSTRUCTION AND UROLITHIASIS

Urinary tract obstruction

Any obstruction in the urinary tract predisposes to UTI and stone formation. Obstruction in the urinary tract can be unilateral or bilateral, complete or incomplete, and of gradual or sudden onset. If the blockage is unrelieved permanent renal atrophy occurs. The following imaging techniques are useful in the diagnosis of urinary tract obstruction as follows:

- Dilatation of the urinary tract may be demonstrated on ultrasound.
- DTPA (diethylenetriamine pentaacetic acid) renography can confirm any functional obstruction.
- Intravenous urography (IVU) will demonstrate anatomical and functional obstruction, but can only be used in the absence of renal failure.
- Retrograde pyelography may be required in some cases.

Careful imaging of the renal tract is essential to determine the site and cause of obstruction (see Chapter 8).

Causes of urinary obstruction

Fig. 10.3 shows the sites of obstruction in the urinary tract.

Congenital abnormalities

These include:

- Urethral strictures.
- Meatal strictures.
- Bladder neck obstruction.
- Ureteropelvic obstruction or stenosis.

Mechanical obstruction of the meatus and urethra only occurs in boys. Severe vesico-ureteric reflux will cause dilatation of the upper renal tract without obstruction.

Tumours

These are mainly large obstuctive masses in the urinary tract (e.g. carcinoma of the pelvis, ureter, bladder, prostate). The external pressure from gynaecological tumours in women on the ureters (i.e. cancer of the cervix) can also cause an obstruction.

Calculi

Renal stones can cause urinary obstruction.

Pregnancy

The high levels of progesterone in pregnancy relax smooth muscle fibres in the renal pelvis and ureters and cause a dysfunctional obstruction. There may also be external compression from the pressure of the enlarging fetus on the ureters.

Hyperplastic lesions

The most common hyperplastic lesion causing urinary obstruction is benign prostatic hypertrophy (BPH).

Inflammation

Any inflammation in the lower urinary tract will cause an obstruction (e.g. urethritis, ureteritis, prostatitis, retroperitoneal fibrosis).

Neurogenic disorders

These result from:

- Congenital anomalies affecting the spinal cord (e.g. spina bifida).
- External pressure on the cord or lumbar nerve roots (e.g. meningioma, lumbar disk prolapse).
- Following trauma to the spinal cord.

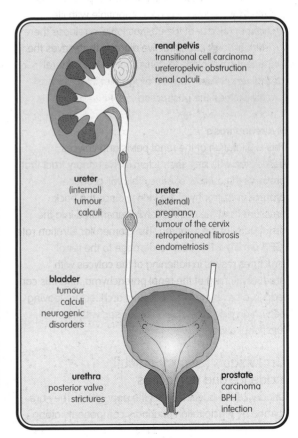

renal pelvis
transitional cell carcinoma
ureteropelvic obstruction
renal calculi

ureter
(internal)
tumour
calculi

ureter
(external)
pregnancy
tumour of the cervix
retroperitoneal fibrosis
endometriosis

bladder
tumour
calculi
neurogenic
disorders

urethra
posterior valve
strictures

prostate
carcinoma
BPH
infection

Fig. 10.3 Sites of obstruction in the urinary tract.

Presentation of urinary obstruction

This depends upon the site and timing of the obstruction:

- An acute, sudden, and complete obstruction in the ureters (e.g. due to a stone) will cause renal colic, which is excruciatingly painful. If unilateral, renal failure will not result.
- An insidious urethral obstruction such as a tumour in the bladder or prostatic hypertrophy will present with bladder distension and related symptoms including hesitancy, terminal dribbling, poor urine flow, and a sense of incomplete emptying.
- A unilateral and partial obstruction causing a hydroureter or hydronephrosis may not be apparent for many years since renal function is maintained by the unaffected kidney.
- A bilateral and partial obstruction presents with nocturia and polyuria due to tubular cell dysfunction and therefore diminished ability to concentrate urine. Other manifestations include renal stones, salt wasting, distal renal tubular acidosis, and hypertension.
- A bilateral and complete obstruction presents as anuria or oliguria. It is not compatible with life without release of the obstruction. On release there is massive post-obstructive diuresis that leaves the patient susceptible to dehydration. Any general malaise or fever may be a sign that infection has complicated the obstruction.

Hydronephrosis

This is dilatation of the renal pelvis and calyces associated with any obstruction in the urinary tract that prevents the outflow of urine. This will produce progressive atrophy of the kidney since the back pressure from the obstruction is transmitted into the distal parts of the nephron. The glomerular filtration rate (GFR) declines. Progressive damage to the renal structures results in flattening of the calyces with gradual thinning of the renal parenchyma, and this can lead to a complete loss of normal architecture leaving behind a cystic thin-walled fibrous sac with no functional capacity.

Urolithiasis (urinary calculi)

Incidence and risk factors

Urinary calculi affect 1–5% of the population. They are formed by precipitation of urinary components along

with a small core of organic material. The factors influencing stone formation include:

- Increased urinary concentration of a substance as a result of high plasma levels (e.g. calcium and urate) or abnormal tubular function (e.g. calcium and cysteine).
- Absence of inhibiting substances (e.g. citrate and phosphate).
- Acidic urinary pH.
- Urinary stasis or obstruction.

The calculi can form anywhere along the urinary tract, but tend to appear most commonly as multiple stones in the renal pelvis. Occasionally a calculus can grow to take up the shape of the renal pelvis (staghorn calculus). The process by which the stones are formed requires initiation by a core of mucoproteins or urates (nucleation); there is then a progressive increase in stone size (aggregation) due to deposition of the main components of the stone. Fig. 10.4 lists the different types of stone and their frequency.

Presentation

The clinical presentation includes:

- Renal colic due to the increase in peristalsis in the ureters when a small stone passes down towards the bladder, obstructing the lumen. This is an exquisitely painful condition, which is described as 'worse than the pain of childbirth'.
- A continuous dull ache in the loins.
- Recurrent and untreatable UTIs.

Different types of renal stone and their frequency	
Type	**Frequency (%)**
calcium-containing stones: • calcium oxalate • calcium phosphate	60–70 10–15
complex triple stones (magnesium, aluminium, phosphate)	15
uric acid stones	5
cysteine stones	1–2

Fig. 10.4 Different types of renal stone and their frequency.

Treatment

Management involves adequate analgesia and a high fluid intake. Stones less than 0.5 cm in width usually pass spontaneously and any larger stones require intervention. Treatment options include:

- Percutaneous surgery involving endoscopic removal of the stone.
- Extracorporeal lithotripsy in which shockwaves are used to fragment the calculi into small pieces which will then pass.

Prevention of renal stones includes:

- A high fluid intake to produce a dilute urine.
- Therapy aimed at correcting the metabolic abnormality.

○ **Discuss the causes of urinary tract obstruction and the various types of presentation.**

○ **What is urolithiasis and what factors may promote its development? Outline the main types of stone and the characteristic symptoms they produce.**

INFLAMMATION OF THE URINARY TRACT

Ureteritis

This is inflammation of the ureter and may occur in UTI. Persistent or recurrent infection leads to chronic inflammation in which there are two reaction patterns:

- Ureteritis folliculitis—as a result of lymphocytic aggregation beneath the epithelium there is elevation of the mucosal surface and a fine granular appearance is seen.
- Ureteritis cystica—multiple small cysts (1–5 mm) project into the lumen. The cysts are thin walled and contain clear fluid. The cysts develop from fibrosed clumps of epithelial cells on the surface of the ureteric mucosa.

Cystitis

This is inflammation of the urinary bladder and is common in UTI. The aetiology and predisposing factors were discussed with UTI (see Chapter 9). The pathogens that cause cystitis are:

- Most commonly *Escherichia coli* and *Proteus* followed by *Enterobacter*.
- *Candida albicans* in patients on long-term antibiotics.
- *Cryptococcus* species in people who are immunosuppressed.
- *Schistosoma*—this is an important causative agent in Middle Eastern countries.
- *Mycobacterium tuberculosis*—tuberculous cystitis is usually indicative of tuberculosis in the upper urinary tract.

Sterile cystis can be caused by radiation damage, drugs, and instrumentation.

Cystitis may be acute or chronic. The most serious complication is pyelonephritis.

Acute cystitis

In acute cystitis the mucosa becomes hyperaemic and this is sometimes associated with an exudate. There are various forms:

- Haemorrhagic cystitis—occurs if the hyperaemia becomes excessive and involves some bleeding.
- Exudative cystitis—the term given when there are yellow areas of fibrinous exudate on the mucosa.
- Suppurative cystitis—characterized by an accumulation of large quantities of exudate.
- Ulcerative cystitis—the term for large areas of ulceration in the bladder mucosa.
- Gangrenous cystitis—the most serious form and due to ischaemia, which results in areas of black necrotic bladder mucosa.

Chronic cystitis

This disorder is due to recurrent or persistent infection of the bladder. The presence of chronic infection leads to fibrous thickening and therefore loss of the elasticity of the bladder wall; elasticity is vital to the bladder's function of urine storage and contraction during micturition.

Presentation and treatment

The classic symptoms of all types of cystitis are:

- Urgency and frequency of micturition.
- Dysuria.
- Lower abdominal pain and tenderness.

There may be associated systemic signs of fever, general malaise, and rigors.

Treatment of cystitis consists in a 3–5 day course of antibiotics; a high fluid intake is advised. If there is recurrent infection investigations should be carried out.

Other types of cystitis

Interstitial cystitis

This is a special form of cystitis. It has an unknown cause and since it is often associated with SLE it is thought to be an autoimmune condition. It has a much higher incidence in women than in men. It may also result from recurrent and persistent infection that results in fibrosis of all the layers of the bladder wall. There is often localized ulceration of the mucosa.

Malakoplakia vesicae

This is a very rare form of cystitis, but it is important because it can mimic a tumour. It is characterized by the formation of plaques on the mucous membrane of the bladder and ureters. These plaques are inflammatory, soft, yellow, 3–5 cm in diameter, and prone to ulceration. On histology the plaques are found to contain foamy macrophages with a granular cytoplasm containing Michaelis–Gutmann bodies and chronic inflammatory cells. The incidence of malakoplakia is increased in renal transplant patients.

Schistosomiasis (bilharzia)

Schistosomiasis is an infection seen commonly worldwide, although it is rare in the UK. It is endemic in the Middle East, Africa, the Far East, and parts of South America. The pathogen is a blood fluke (*Schistosoma haematobium*), which causes chronic irritation of the transitional cells of the bladder as it settles in the bladder to lay eggs. Humans are infected by the cercarial phase of the parasite released by freshwater snails. Penetration through intact skin allows entry into the venous system from where the schistosomes migrate to the liver and bladder. The eggs are excreted into local water supplies and the cycle is completed through freshwater snails (Fig. 10.5).

People infected with cercariae may present with an itchy papular rash accompanied by myalgia, abdominal pain, and headache. The most common presentation of infection with *S. haematobium* is recurrent haematuria.

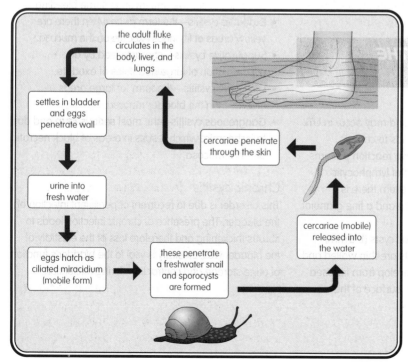

Fig. 10.5 Infestation with *S. haematobium*.

the adult fluke circulates in the body, liver, and lungs

settles in bladder and eggs penetrate wall

urine into fresh water

eggs hatch as ciliated miracidium (mobile form)

these penetrate a freshwater snail and sporocysts are formed

cercariae (mobile) released into the water

cercariae penetrate through the skin

Eventually, obstruction within the urinary tract, bladder calcification, and renal failure occur.

Diagnosis involves detection of the eggs in the urine or enzyme-linked immunosorbent assay (ELISA) for evidence of a response to infection.

Treatment consists in praziquantel given once daily.

Urethral inflammation

The commonest pathogens are *E. coli* and *Proteus*. Ascending infection including cystitis, ureteritis and pyelitis can result.

Acute inflammation of the urethra can occur as a result of infection with a sexually transmitted disease (e.g. *N. gonorrhoea* or *Chlamydia trachomatis*) (see Crash Course! Endocrine and Reproductive System for full coverage). Urethritis in association with conjunctivitis and arthritis can occur in Reiter's disease.

Discuss the following inflammatory conditions of the urinary tract:
○ **Urethritis.**
○ **Cystitis.**
○ **Schistosomiasis.**

NEOPLASTIC DISEASE OF THE URINARY TRACT

Tumours of the ureters
Benign tumours of the ureter
Small benign tumours of the ureter are derived from blood vessels, lymphatics, and smooth muscle. A fibroepithelial polyp is a small mass that projects into the lumen. It consists of a clump of vascular connective tissue beneath the ureteric mucosa.

Malignant tumours of the ureters
Primary malignancies are very rare and metastatic disease is relatively more common in the ureters. Malignant tumours arise from the transitional epithelium that lines the ureters and most of the urinary tract. They are usually clinically silent for many years and are found in 60–70 year olds. They eventually present as a partial and unilateral obstruction as the ureteric lumen is occluded. They often occur in association with multiple tumours of the bladder and renal pelvis (synchronous tumours of the uroepithelium).

Tumours of the bladder
Metaplasia
The transitional cell lining (urothelium) of the bladder can undergo metaplastic changes during any period of infection or inflammation as a result of stones, drugs, and radiation. There are three types of metaplasia:
- Squamous metaplasia—occurs in areas of long-term chronic inflammation in exstrophy of the bladder, bladder calculi, and schistosomiasis and predisposes to squamous cell carcinoma.
- Intestinal or glandular metaplasia—associated with chronic cystitis and leads to the formation of slit-like glands of columnar epithelium.
- Nephrogenic metaplasia—rare, consists of multiple projections of the mucosal lining, and must be differentiated from adenocarcinoma.

Benign tumours of the bladder
These are very rare and make up 2–3% of bladder epithelial tumours. Transitional cell papilloma may be the first stage (grade I) of transitional cell carcinoma. These papillomas are often multiple and are found all over the mucosal lining. They are small projections 0.5–2.0 cm in length. They have a branched structure and are attached to the mucosa by a small stalk with a fibrovascular core covered in urothelium.

The other benign lesions are inverted papillomas. These consist of solitary nodules in the mucosa and measure 1–3 cm in diameter.

Transitional cell carcinomas
These are malignant tumours that arise from the transitional cell epithelium that lines the bladder and make up over 90% of bladder epithelial cell tumours. The number of cases is increasing. They are uncommon under 50 years of age. The male to female ratio is 4:1.

Presentation
The commonest presentation of any tumour of the bladder is painless haematuria. This is often accompanied by symptoms of a UTI (i.e. dysuria, frequency, and urgency). Presenting symptoms may also arise from local invasion of the tumour causing ureteric obstruction. Predisposing factors include smoking, exposure to chemicals in the rubber industry (e.g. naphthylamine and benzidine) and analgesic abuse.

157

Pathology

There are different morphological types of transitional cell tumours (Fig. 10.6):

- Papillary tumour (70%)—exophytic lesion consisting of delicate fronds covered in a thick layer of urothelium branching off a stalk that attaches it to the mucosa.
- Sessile (flat) tumour—plaques of thickened mucosa with a well-defined border and often noninvasive.

Both these types of tumour can be *in situ* or invasive.

- In-situ carcinomas are the precursors of the invasive tumours.
- Invasive tumours infiltrate the basement membrane of the bladder mucosa and the lamina propria and can penetrate adjacent structures once through the mucosal wall.

Transitional cell carcinomas can be graded according to the degree of cellular atypia on histology:

- Grade I—there is an increase in the number of epithelial cell layers (over seven) and there is some cell atypia.
- Grade II—there is an increase in cell layers (over 10) and there is a large variation in cell size and in nucleus shape and size.
- Grade III—the cells have no resemblance to their cells of origin and there is a loss of connections between the cells causing them to fragment.

There is a continuous pattern of growth from the relatively benign well-differentiated papillary growths (grade I) to the formation of solid plaque-like anaplastic tumours (grade III) as the carcinoma progresses. There

is a high rate of correlation between the clinical staging and the grade. Grade III tumours are often ulcerated and have penetrated though the bladder muscle wall and are associated with the worst prognosis.

Many of the carcinomas show areas of squamous or glandular metaplasia and if the extent is over 5% they are called mixed tumours.

The current system used for the staging of transitional cell tumours is the TNM system (Fig. 10.7). This staging system recognizes both local and distant tumour spread:

- Local spread involves invasion into the bladder wall and extension to adjacent structures.
- Distant spread includes spread to the regional lymph nodes and metastases in the liver and lungs.

Histological examination is vital to determine whether the muscle is involved. The distinction between the lamina propria invasion and submucosal invasion has recently been correlated with the prognosis. There is also a correlation between the stage and the grade of the tumours. Staging is a useful predictor of prognosis in these tumours.

Most of the tumours are situated on the posterior and lateral walls of the bladder, and they are often multiple, suggesting that the entire epithelium is unstable due to exposure to the carcinogen.

Diagnosis, treatment, and prognosis

Diagnosis is made by cytological examination of the urine to check for the presence of malignant cells and by cystoscopy of the lower urinary tract.

Treatment depends upon the stage and differentiation of the tumour. Treatment includes cystodiathermy, resection of the tumour with close follow-up, radiotherapy, chemotherapy, and cystectomy.

The average 5-year survival rate is 80% if the bladder wall is not involved and 5% if there is local metastasis on presentation.

Squamous cell carcinoma

These usually arise in areas of squamous metaplasia of the bladder mucosa and account for <10% of bladder carcinomas. The predisposing factors include bladder extrophy, calculi, and schistosomiasis. These cause chronic irritation to the transitional cells of the bladder, which leads to squamous metaplasia, which becomes

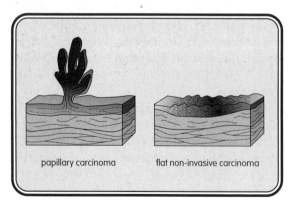

papillary carcinoma   flat non-invasive carcinoma

Fig. 10.6 Two morphological types of tumour.

dysplastic resulting in carcinoma *in situ*. This then progresses to invasive squamous cell carcinoma.

The tumours are solid, ulcerative, invasive, and fungating masses, and are often very extensive on discovery. Their prognosis is worse than that of transitional cell carcinoma.

Adenocarcinoma

This is rare in the bladder and usually arises from urachal remnants, metaplasia of the transitional epithelium or cystitis cystica. They are most common in the apex of the bladder.

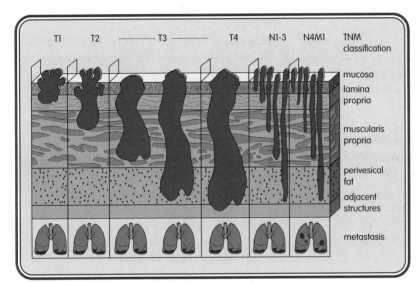

Fig. 10.7 TNM staging system for transitional cell carcinoma of bladder. T staging decribes tumour invasion of the tissue layers. N staging describes degree of spread to the lymph nodes: 1 = local nodes; 2 = distant nodes below the diaphragm; 3 = distant nodes on both sides of the diaphragm. M staging describes the presence or absence of metastases: 0 = none; 1 = present. (From Management of Urologic Disorders by Dr RR Bahnson. Mosby Year-Book, 1994.

o **What are the three types of metaplastic change that occur in the bladder?**
o **Discuss transitional cell tumours noting their incidence and presentation, predisposing factors, and different morphological types, grading, and staging.**
o **What proportion of bladder carcinomas are squamous cell carcinomas?**
o **What are the predisposing factors leading to invasive carcinoma?**

DISORDERS OF THE PROSTATE

Prostatitis

There are three subgroups of inflammation of the prostate.

Acute prostatitis

The main pathogens involved are *E. coli*, *Proteus,* and *Staphylococcus,* and sexually transmitted pathogens including *Chlamydia trachomatis* and gonorrhoea. Inflammation may be focal or diffuse. Infection is usually spread from an acute infection in the urethra or bladder due to:

- Intraprostatic reflux of urine.
- Intraprostatic catheterization.
- Endoscopy of the urethra.

Rarely, acute prostatitis is caused by seeding of a bloodborne infection.

On histology there is an acute inflammatory infiltrate of neutrophils and damaged cells, often resulting in abscess formation.

Patients present with:

- General symptoms such as malaise, rigors, and fever.
- Local symptoms of difficulty in passing urine, dysuria, and perineal tenderness.

On rectal examination the prostate is soft, tender, and enlarged. Diagnosis is confirmed by the clinical findings and by a positive urine culture.

Chronic prostatitis

This disorder is the result of inadequately treated acute disease. This may be because some antibiotics have a very poor ability to penetrate the prostate. There is often a typical history of recurrent prostatic and urinary tract infections. The causative pathogens are the same as for acute prostatic infection.

Patients present with dysuria and low back and perineal pain, though some cases are asymptomatic and the disease appears with no preceding acute phase.

Chronic prostatitis is a very difficult condition to diagnose and treat. Diagnosis is confirmed by:

- The histological appearance of neutrophils, plasma cells, and lymphocytes.
- A positive culture from a sample of prostatic secretion.

Tuberculosis is another cause of chronic infection and is associated with tuberculosis in the kidneys or epididymis. On histology there are focal areas of caseation and giant-cell infiltrates.

Chronic non-bacterial prostatitis

This is the most common type of prostatitis and results in enlargement of the prostate, which can obstruct the urethra. The pathogen involved is *Chlamydia trachomatis*. Often there is no history of recurrent UTIs.

Presentation is similar to that of chronic prostatits and on histology there is fibrosis as a result of chronic inflammation.

Diagnosis is confirmed by the presence of 15 white blood cells per high power field and repeated negative bacterial cultures.

Benign prostatic hypertrophy (BPH)

Incidence

BPH is the commonest disorder of the prostate and occurs in men over 60 years of age. It is a non-neoplastic enlargement of the gland and the cause is unknown although it is seen in 80% of 80-year-old men.

Presentation

Symptoms of BPH are due to the pressure of the enlarging gland on the urethra passing through it and the swelling of the periurethral gland, which affects the bladder sphincter mechanism. Patients present with:

- Difficulty or hesitancy in starting to urinate.
- A poor stream.
- Dribbling post-micturition.

These symptoms are referred to as prostatism.

Untreated BPH can present with acute retention of urine, which is accompanied by a distended and tender bladder. Chronic retention is associated with nocturnal overflow incontinence and a distended non-tender bladder.

Examination must include abdominal examination for an enlarged bladder and a rectal examination for the prostate, which is firm, smooth, and rubbery.

Pathology

There is hyperplasia of both the lateral lobes and the periurethral glands, which lie posterior to the urethra (this is referred to as median lobe enlargement) leading to distortion of the urethra and therefore obstruction of bladder outflow. Within the prostate there are solid nodules of fibromuscular material and cystic regions. On histology there is hyperplasia of:

- Stroma (smooth muscle and fibrous tissue).
- The glandular components of the prostatic tissue, often with areas of infarction and necrosis.

Complications

The complications of benign prostatic hypertrophy result from prolonged obstruction to urine flow. There is compensatory hypertrophy of the bladder as a result of the high pressures that develop within the bladder (Fig. 10.8).

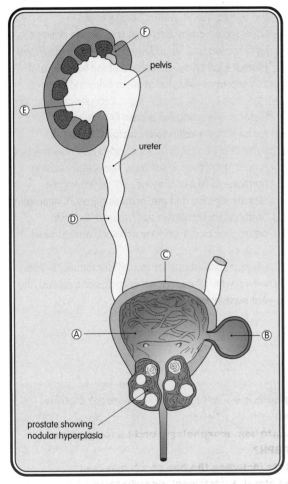

Fig. 10.8 Complications of benign prostatic hyperplasia. (A) Bands of thickened smooth muscle fibre cause trabeculation of the bladder wall. (B) Diverticula may develop on the external surface of the bladder. (C) Dilatation of the bladder once the muscle becomes hypotonic. (D) Formation of hydroureters resulting in the reflux of urine up to the renal pelvis. (E) Bilateral hydronephrosis. (F) Kidney infection, stones, calculi, and failure.

Treatment

Surgical treatment consists in transurethral resection of the prostate (TURP), which is quick and safe with a low mortality and a good success rate.

Medical managemnet involves the treatment of prostatic symptoms with α-blockers (which relax smooth muscle and improve urinary flow rate) and anti-androgens such as finasteride. Finasteride is a 5α-reductase inhibitor that prevents the conversion of testosterone to the more potent androgen dihydrotestosterone. Dihydrotestosterone promotes growth and enlargement of the prostate; inhibition of its production leads to a decrease in prostate volume and an improvement in urinary flow rate and obstructive symptoms.

Carcinoma of the prostate

Incidence and risk factors

Prostate cancer is the third commonest cancer in men after cancer of the lung and stomach. It accounts for 8% of all cancers in men. It is a disease of elderly men, occurring in one in ten men of 70 years of age. It is rare under 55 years of age and has a strong hereditary component.

The aetiology is unknown, but there is a link between androgenic hormones and tumour growth. The lesions are most commonly found in the periphery of the posterior part of the prostate compared with the more central and lateral location of BPH—these areas have different embryological origins and often both conditions coexist.

Presentation

Patients present with symptoms of UTI, prostatism, or metastatic disease in the bone causing bone pain. Carcinoma may be found coincidentally in autopsies of elderly men who were asymptomatic. About 25% of the patients have symptoms of metastatic disease on presentation.

Pathology

The tumours form a range of morphological subtypes ranging from well-differentiated single nodules to anaplastic and diffuse involvement of all lobes of the gland. The Gleeson classification is used to grade the tumours on histological appearance. Grade 1 is a well-differentiated tumour composed of uniform tumour cells while grade 5 is an anaplastic diffuse tumour with cells showing great variation in their structure and a high mitotic rate.

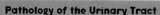
Spread takes place by:
- Local invasion of adjacent structures including the bladder and ureters.
- Lymphatic spread.
- Haematogenous seeding of tumour cells to the bones of the spine and pelvis and occasionally to the lungs and liver.

Stage is determined by the universal TNM system:
- T_1—no tumour is palpable.
- T_2—the tumour is confined to the prostate.
- T_3—there is extension of the tumour beyond the prostatic capsule.
- T_4—the tumour has fixed the adjacent structures.

T is tumour classification. The prefix of N is used to describe the lymph node involvement and M, metastases.

Diagnosis

On rectal examination the prostate feels hard and irregular. Prostatic ultrasound may be helpful in defining a prostatic mass. A raised prostatic specific antigen (PSA) level in the blood is indicative of prostatic cancer; however, a normal result does not exclude the presence of malignant disease. Serum prostatic acid phosphatase is also raised, especially if there are metastases. Levels of PSA and acid phosphatase can be used to monitor response to treatment.

Radiographs and bone scans are used in the staging of the disease. Typical osteosclerotic lesions on radiographs and increased isotope uptake on bone scans are seen in metastatic disease of prostatic carcinoma (see Chapter 8).

Treatment and prognosis

Treatment options include surgery, hormone therapy, and radiotherapy. Before the start of any treatment a histological diagnosis of prostatic carcinoma is required. The specimen is taken by transurethral or transrectal biopsy. Treatment depends upon the size of the tumour:
- If the lesion is confined within the capsule of the gland the treatment of choice is surgical resection of the prostate (prostatectomy). TURP may also be required in advanced metastatic disease to relieve the symptoms of urethral obstruction.
- Local radiotherapy is used in very elderly patients who are too unfit to undergo surgery. It is also used to treat local or distant spread of the tumour, and can provide useful palliation for bony metastases.
- Hormone manipulation—testosterone is an important factor in promoting the growth of the tumours, and removal of the testes (orchidectomy) is often a successful treatment for more advanced disease, but is now rarely used. Luteinizing hormone-releasing hormone (LHRH) analogues (e.g. buserelin) are equally effective and are increasingly used. Alternative hormone manipulation can be used (e.g. with oestrogens and antiandrogens such as flutamide).

The 5-year survival rate for grade 1 tumour is 75–90%. However, when there is local or metastatic spread, the 5-year survival falls to 30–45%.

- **What are the three types of inflammation affecting the prostate? Outline the causes of infection and presentation of each.**
- **Define BPH and outline its presentation, morphology, and histology. What are the major complications of BPH?**
- **Discuss carcinoma of the prostate including the age group affected, presentation, morphology of the gland, histological classification, and staging.**

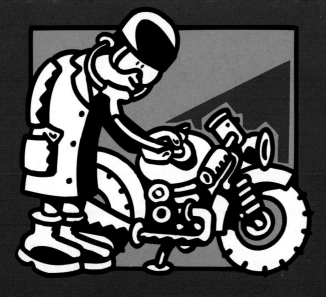

SELF-ASSESSMENT

Indicate whether each answer is true or false.

1. **Potassium excretion by the kidney can be modified by alterations in:**

(a) The electric profile of the distal nephron (i.e. degree of electronegativity of tubule lumen compared to that of blood).
(b) Urine flow rate.
(c) Urinary Na^+ concentration.
(d) Urine pH.
(e) Plasma aldosterone concentration.

2. **Subjects A and B are 70 kg males. Subject A drinks 2 L of distilled water and Subject B drinks 2 L of isotonic NaCl. As a result, subject B will have:**

(a) Greater change in ICF volume.
(b) Higher positive free water clearance.
(c) Greater change in plasma osmolarity.
(d) Higher urine osmolarity.
(e) Higher urine flow rate.

3. **A woman with a history of severe diarrhoea has the following arterial blood values—pH 7.25, pCO_2 3.2 kPa, HCO_3^- 10 mmol/L. The correct diagnosis is:**

(a) Normal acid–base status.
(b) Metabolic acidosis.
(c) Metabolic alkalosis.
(d) Respiratory acidosis.
(e) Respiratory alkalosis.

4. **Match the following blood gas results with one of the clinical situations listed below—pH 7.45, pCO_2 3.3 kPa, pO_2 8.0 kPa:**

(a) Hyperventilation.
(b) Diabetic ketoacidosis.
(c) Pyloric stenosis.
(d) Mild asthma.
(e) Chronic obstructive airways disease (COAD).

5. **Match the following blood gas results with one of the clinical situations listed below—pH 7.5, pCO_2 3.7 kPa, pO_2 14.4 kPa:**

(a) Hyperventilation.
(b) Diabetic ketoacidosis.
(c) Pyloric stenosis.
(d) Mild asthma.
(e) COAD.

6. **Match the following blood gas results with one of the clinical situations listed below—pH 7.15, pCO_2 4.1 kPa, pO_2 13.3 kPa:**

(a) Hyperventilation.
(b) Diabetic ketoacidosis.
(c) Pyloric stenosis.
(d) Mild asthma.
(e) COAD.

7. **Match the following blood gas results with one of the clinical situations listed below—pH 7.34, pCO_2 7.3 kPa, pO_2 8.8 kPa:**

(a) Hyperventilation.
(b) Diabetic ketoacidosis.
(c) Pyloric stenosis.
(d) Mild asthma.
(e) COAD.

8. **Match the following blood gas results with one of the clinical situations listed below—pH 7.53, pCO_2 42, pO_2 13.3 kPa:**

(a) Hyperventilation.
(b) Diabetic ketoacidosis.
(c) Pyloric stenosis.
(d) Mild asthma.
(e) COAD.

9. **Glomerular filtration rate is:**

(a) Altered by eating a high protein meal.
(b) Accurately measured by p-aminohuppuric acid (PAH) clearance.
(c) About 20% of plasma flow.
(d) Modified by the macula densa.
(e) Is about 180 L per day.

10. **The anion gap:**

(a) Is normally 20–25 mmol/L.
(b) Increased after methanol ingestion.
(c) Is normal after ethylene glycol ingestion.
(d) May be abnormal in chronic uraemia.
(e) Is affected by lactic acidosis.

11. **Plasma creatinine concentration:**

(a) Is never affected by diet.
(b) Is a sensitive guide to mild renal impairment.
(c) Depends upon weight.
(d) Is disproportionately increased compared to urea in rhabdomyolysis.
(e) Reflects glomerulation filtration.

12. Which of the following would increase glomerular filtration rate (GFR)?

(a) Hyperproteinaemia.
(b) A ureteral stone.
(c) Dilatation of the afferent arteriole.
(d) Dilatation of the efferent arteriole.
(e) Constriction of the efferent arteriole.

13. Which of the following would distinguish a healthy person with severe water deprivation from a person with syndrome of inappropriate antidiuretic hormone (SIADH)?

(a) Clearance of free water.
(b) Urine osmolarity.
(c) Plasma osmolarity.
(d) Circulating levels of ADH.
(e) Effective treatment with demeclocyline.

14. Acute renal failure (ARF):

(a) May be caused by Wegener's granulomatosis.
(b) May be irreversible.
(c) Is always associated with abnormalities on urine dipstick.
(d) Is a recognized complication of non-steroidal anti-inflammatory drug (NSAID) use.
(e) Can be effectively treated by dopamine infusion.

15. Nephrotic syndrome can be caused by:

(a) Gold.
(b) Penicillamine.
(c) Staphylococcal infection.
(d) Captopril.
(e) Paracetamol.

16. The following can be features of the nephritic syndrome:

(a) Oliguria.
(b) Low blood pressure.
(c) Haematuria.
(d) Decreased serum urea and creatinine.
(e) Evidence of a recent streptococcal infection.

17. Urinary tract obstruction:

(a) Is most often congenital in children.
(b) Is most common in men over 60 years of age.
(c) Is confined to the ureter.
(d) Can present as renal colic.
(e) Does not predispose to infection.

18. Diabetic nephropathy:

(a) Is more frequent in non-insulin-dependent diabetes mellitus (NIDDM) than insulin-dependent diabetes mellitus (IDDM).
(b) Is rare before 20 years of age.

(c) Can present as the nephrotic syndrome.
(d) Once present usually progresses to end-stage renal failure.
(e) Is characterized by microhaematuria.

19. Distribution of water:

(a) Intracellular fluid (ICF) accounts for one-third of total body water (TBW).
(b) The major cation of ICF is K^+.
(c) Extracellular fluid (ECF) is comprised of interstitial fluid, plasma, and transcellular fluid.
(d) The major anions of ECF are Cl^- and HCO_3^-.
(e) Inulin is used to measure ICF.

20. Adrenocortical insufficiency:

(a) Results in decreased osmolarity of ECF.
(b) Results in increased ECF volume.
(c) Results in increased haematocrit.
(d) Can occur after prolonged corticosteroid administration.
(e) Results in hypokalaemia.

21. Thiazide diuretics:

(a) Cause metabolic acidosis.
(b) Cause hyperuricaemia.
(c) Cause glucose intolerance.
(d) Cause hypocalcaemia.
(e) Are used in the treatment of angina.

22. The following statements are correct:

(a) The kidneys receive approximately 20% of the cardiac output.
(b) In healthy young adults approximately 130 ml/min of protein-free filtrate is formed at the glomeruli.
(c) Non-protein bound drug of molecular weight less than 66 kDa passes into the filtrate.
(d) Potentially saturable mechanisms for active secretion of both acids and bases exist in the proximal tubule.
(e) Low lipid solubility favours tubular reabsorption.

23. The following can impair renal function:

(a) Naproxen.
(b) Ranitidine.
(c) Iodine-containing contrast media.
(d) Captopril.
(e) Amphotericin B.

24. To maintain normal H^+ balance, total daily excretion of H^+ should equal the daily:

(a) Fixed acid production plus fixed acid ingestion.
(b) HCO_3^- excretion.
(c) HCO_3^- filtered load.
(d) Titratable acid excretion.
(e) Filtered load of H^+.

25. The following are secreted by the proximal tubule:

(a) Sodium.
(b) Potassium.
(c) Glucose.
(d) Bicarbonate.
(e) Water.

26. Production of urea is increased by:

(a) Old age.
(b) A low protein diet.
(c) Tetracycline.
(d) Glucocorticosteroid therapy.
(e) Surgery.

27. Renin release is controlled by:

(a) Osmotic concentration in the distal tubule.
(b) Pressure changes in the efferent arterioles.
(c) Parasympathetic tone.
(d) Local prostaglandin release.
(e) Chloride concentration in the distal tubule.

28. The following statements about resting renal blood flow are correct:

(a) The glomerular filtration pressure is about 80 mmHg.
(b) 10 000 nephrons receive 1.2 L of blood/min.
(c) The glomerular capillaries are supplied by the afferent arterioles.
(d) The afferent arterioles supply blood directly to the distal tubules.
(e) The blood supply of the medulla arises from the efferent arterioles.

29. Erythropoietin secretion may be increased by:

(a) Polycystic renal disease.
(b) Benign renal cysts.
(c) Renal cell carcinoma.
(d) Loss of renal substance.
(e) Nephrotic syndrome.

30. Glomerulonephritis:

(a) Affects both kidneys.
(b) May be caused by immune complex disease.
(c) Is always the result of deposition of anti-glomerular basement membrane (anti-GBM) antibody.
(d) Is always associated with pyelonephritis.
(e) Is associated with red cell casts on urine microscopy.

31. Life-threatening complications of acute glomerulonephritis include:

(a) Hypertensive encephalopathy.
(b) Pulmonary oedema.
(c) Uraemia.
(d) Epilepsy.
(e) Stroke.

32. The renal excretion of water is dependent upon:

(a) GFR.
(b) Reabsorption of solute in the proximal tubule.
(c) Concentration of ADH.
(d) Normal functioning distal convoluted tubule.
(e) Solute concentration in the thick ascending limb of the loop of Henle.

33. Factors that increase the formation of urinary tract stones (urolithiasis) include:

(a) Cushing's syndrome.
(b) Dehydration.
(c) Hypocalcaemia.
(d) Urinary tract infection (UTI).
(e) Pregnancy.

34. Clinical features of urinary tract stones are:

(a) Asymptomatic.
(b) Haematuria.
(c) Renal colic.
(d) UTI.
(e) Urinary tract obstruction.

35. The following statements about potassium metabolism are true:

(a) Intracellular potassium concentration is 150 mmol/L.
(b) Cellular uptake of potassium is decreased by insulin.
(c) Normal dietary intake is about 2–3 g/day.
(d) 20% of daily intake is excreted in the urine.
(e) Depletion of potassium is associated with metabolic alkalosis.

36. Predisposing factors in UTI are:

(a) Vesico-ureteric reflux (VUR).
(b) Diabetes mellitus.
(c) Postmenopausal lack of oestrogen.
(d) Neurogenic bladder.
(e) Structural urinary tract abnormality.

37. Causes of urinary tract obstruction include:

(a) Urethral strictures.
(b) Retroperitoneal fibrosis.
(c) Prostate cancer.
(d) Renal stones.
(e) Pregnancy.

38. Urinary tract obstruction can present with:

(a) Renal colic.
(b) Hydronephrosis.
(c) Polyuria.
(d) Anuria.
(e) Stress incontinence.

39. Causes of acute tubular necrosis (ATN) include:

(a) Severe burns.
(b) Gentamicin.
(c) Vitamin A.
(d) Gold salts.
(e) Paracetamol.

40. ATN:

(a) Can initially present with oliguria.
(b) Is reversible with supportive treatment.
(c) Is associated with hypokalaemia.
(d) Is never associated with sepsis.
(e) Can be toxin related.

41. Management of chronic renal failure includes:

(a) A high protein diet.
(b) Regular checks on parathyroid hormones.
(c) Antihypertensive treatment.
(d) Correction of anaemia with erythropoietin.
(e) Renal replacement therapy.

42. The following ions have a higher concentration in ECF than in ICF:

(a) Na^+.
(b) K^+.
(c) Cl^-.
(d) HCO_3^-.
(e) Ca^{2+}.

43. The following are causes of metabolic acidosis:

(a) Vomiting.
(b) Diarrhoea.
(c) Chronic renal failure.
(d) Ethylene glycol ingestion.
(e) Hyperaldosteronism.

44. The following cause hyperkalaemia:

(a) Exercise.
(b) Alkalosis.
(c) Treatment with β-agonists (i.e. salbutamol).
(d) Insulin administration.
(e) Decreased serum osmolarity.

45. The right kidney:

(a) Is posteriorly related to the second part of the duodenum.
(b) Lies laterally to the aorta.
(c) Is higher than the left kidney.
(d) Lies anterior to psoas muscle.
(e) Has a colonic impression on its anterior surface.

46. Benign prostatic hypertrophy (BPH):

(a) Occurs most often in men under 60 years of age.
(b) Is associated with median lobe enlargement.
(c) Acute retention requires surgical treatment.
(d) Can metastasize.
(e) Can present with UTI.

47. Renal cell carcinoma:

(a) Is the most common renal tumour in adults.
(b) Can present with bony metastases.
(c) Is associated with a high α-fetoprotein.
(d) Arises from the proximal tubule epithelium.
(e) Has an increased incidence in von Hippel–Lindau disease.

48. In adult polycystic disease of the kidney:

(a) The inheritance is autosomal dominant.
(b) Massive proteinuria is always found.
(c) The diagnosis is compatible with a normal life span.
(d) The cysts involve all parts of the nephron.
(e) There is a recognized association with intracerebral aneurysms.

49. Osmoreceptors:

(a) Detect variations in plasma osmolality.
(b) Are located in the thalamus.
(c) Receive blood supply from the internal carotid artery.
(d) Have no effect on thirst.
(e) Regulate the release of ADH.

50. ADH release is increased by:

(a) Nicotine.
(b) Morphine.
(c) Alcohol.
(d) Barbiturates.
(e) β-blockers.

1. What are the functions of the kidneys?

2. Describe the renal blood supply.

3. Write short notes on the fetal development of the urinary system.

4. Give two examples of how failure of the normal development of renal tract may lead to anatomical abnormalities.

5. Write short notes on the structure of the glomerular filter.

6. Write short notes on the transport processes of the renal tubule.

7. How are the glomerular filtration rate (GFR) and renal blood flow (RBF) measured?

8. What are the age-related changes in RBF and GFR?

9. Discuss the transport of glucose in the proximal tubule and how this correlates with plasma glucose levels.

10. Discuss the reabsorption of bicarbonate ions in the proximal tubule.

11. Draw the adult nephron and label the afferent and efferent arterioles, glomerulus, and tubular segments.

12. Discuss diabetes mellitus and related renal problems.

13. By what mechanism do angiotensin-converting enzyme (ACE) inhibitors decrease hypertension?

14. Write short notes on renal artery stenosis (RAS) and how ACE inhibitors can cause renal impairment in people with RAS?

15. Write short notes on the structure, blood supply, innervation, and functions of the urinary bladder.

16. Write short notes on renal cell carcinoma (RCC).

17. Write short notes on urinary tract obstruction.

18. Write about the anion gap and its indications and interpretation.

19. What are the five main mechanisms of glomerular injury?

20. Write short notes on the complications of benign prostatic hypertrophy.

1. Describe the methods used to measure body fluid compartments including (a) plasma volume, red cell volume, and blood volume, (b) extracellular fluid (ECF), (c) interstitial fluid (ISF), (d) total body water (TBW), (e) transcellular fluid (TCF).

2. Discuss the various anatomical sections of the loop of Henle and how this acts as a countercurrent multiplier.

3. Discuss the actions and side effects of the five classes of diuretics.

4. Write an essay on the management of chronic renal failure.

5. Discuss the causes, symptoms, and signs of the syndrome of inappropriate ADH (SIADH) secretion.

6. Discuss the control of the renin–angiotensin–aldosterone system. What drugs act on this system?

7. Discuss the renal handling of sodium as an example of how filtrate is modified by various aspects of the nephron to produce the excreted product.

8. Discuss the predisposition, presentation, and complications of urinary tract infections.

9. Compare and contrast the reabsorption of salts and water in the proximal convoluted tubule with that in the distal convoluted tubule and cortical collecting duct.

10. Discuss the causes, clinical features, and compensation mechanisms of the following acid–base disturbances: (a) respiratory acidosis, (b) respiratory alkalosis, (c) metabolic acidosis, (d) metabolic alkalosis.

1. (a)T, (b)T, (c)T, (d)T, (e)T

2. (a)F, (b)F, (c)F, (d)T, (e)F

3. (a)F, (b)T, (c)F, (d)F, (e)F

4. (a)F, (b)F, (c)F, (d)T, (e)F

5. (a)T, (b)F, (c)F, (d)F, (e)F

6. (a)F, (b)T, (c)F, (d)F, (e)F

7. (a)F, (b)F, (c)F, (d)F, (e)T

8. (a)F, (b)F, (c)T, (d)F, (e)F

9. (a)T, (b)F, (c)T, (d)T, (e)T

10. (a)F, (b)T, (c)F, (d)T, (e)T

11. (a)F, (b)F, (c)T, (d)T, (e)T

12. (a)F, (b)F, (c)T, (d)F, (e)T

13. (a)F, (b)F, (c)T, (d)F, (e)T

14. (a)T, (b)T, (c)F, (d)T, (e)F

15. (a)T, (b)T, (c)F, (d)T, (e)F

16. (a)T, (b)F, (c)T, (d)F, (e)T

17. (a)T, (b)T, (c)F, (d)T, (e)F

18. (a)F, (b)T, (c)T, (d)T, (e)F

19. (a)F, (b)T, (c)T, (d)T, (e)F

20. (a)T, (b)F, (c)T, (d)T, (e)F

21. (a)F, (b)T, (c)T, (d)F, (e)F

22. (a)T, (b)T, (c)T, (d)T, (e)F

23. (a)T, (b)F, (c)T, (d)T, (e)T

24. (a)T, (b)F, (c)F, (d)F, (e)F

25. (a)F, (b)F, (c)F, (d)F, (e)F

26. (a)F, (b)F, (c)T, (d)T, (e)T

27. (a)T, (b)F, (c)F, (d)T, (e)T

28. (a)F, (b)F, (c)T, (d)F, (e)T

29. (a)T, (b)T, (c)T, (d)F, (e)F

30. (a)T, (b)T, (c)F, (d)F, (e)T

31. (a)T, (b)T, (c)T, (d)F, (e)F

32. (a)T, (b)T, (c)T, (d)T, (e)T

33. (a)T, (b)T, (c)F, (d)T, (e)F

34. (a)T, (b)T, (c)T, (d)T, (e)T

35. (a)T, (b)F, (c)T, (d)F, (e)T

36. (a)T, (b)T, (c)T, (d)T, (e)T

37. (a)T, (b)T, (c)T, (d)T, (e)T

38. (a)T, (b)T, (c)T, (d)T, (e)F

39. (a)T, (b)T, (c)F, (d)F, (e)T

40. (a)T, (b)T, (c)F, (d)F, (e)T

41. (a)F, (b)T, (c)T, (d)T, (e)T

42. (a)T, (b)F, (c)T, (d)T, (e)T

43. (a)F, (b)T, (c)T, (d)T, (e)F

44. (a)T, (b)F, (c)F, (d)F, (e)F

45. (a)T, (b)F, (c)F, (d)T, (e)T

46. (a)F, (b)T, (c)T, (d)F, (e)T

47. (a)T, (b)T, (c)F, (d)T, (e)T

48. (a)T, (b)F, (c)T, (d)T, (e)T

49. (a)T, (b)F, (c)T, (d)F, (e)T

50. (a)T, (b)T, (c)F, (d)T, (e)F

SAQ Answers

1. (a) Regulation of water content, mineral composition, and pH of the body by excreting each substance in an amount adequate to achieve total body balance and maintain normal concentration in the extracellular fluid.
(b) Elimination of metabolic waste products from the blood and their excretion in urine (e.g. urea from protein metabolism, uric acid from nucleic acids, creatinine from muscle creatine).
(c) Removal of foreign chemicals from blood and excretion in urine (e.g. drugs, pesticides, food additives).
(d) Secretion of hormones: erythropoietin to control erythrocyte production; renin to generate angiotensin I from angiotensinogen and so control blood pressure and sodium balance; 1,25-dihydroxyvitamin D3 to influence calcium metabolism.

2. The kidneys receive 20–25% of the total cardiac output (1.2 L/min). The blood enters the kidney via the right and left renal arteries. These branch to form about five interlobar arteries, which divide to form the arcuate arteries located at the junction between the cortex and medulla. The interlobular arteries arise at 90 degrees to the arcuate arteries and pass through the cortex dividing up to form the afferent arterioles, which supply the glomerular capillaries. The efferent arterioles drain blood from the glomerular capillaries acting as portal vessels (i.e. carrying blood from one capillary network to another). In the outer two-thirds of the cortex the efferent arterioles form a network of peritubular capillaries that supply all the cortical parts of the nephron. In the inner third of the cortex the capillaries go on to follow a hairpin course adjacent to the loops of Henle and the collecting ducts down into the medulla. These vessels are known as the vasa recta. The vasa recta and the peritubular capillaries drain into the left and right renal veins and then into the inferior vena cava. Fig. 2.5 shows the microcirculation of the kidney.

3. There are three consecutive systems that form the adult urinary tract—pronephros, mesonephros, and metanephros.
(a) The pronephros develops in the cervical region of the embryo and is rudimentary.
(b) The mesonephros has characteristic excretory units with their own collecting ducts called the mesonephric duct or the wolffian duct. It develops in the thoracic and lumbar regions as the pronephros regresses. It may function for a short time.
(c) The metanephros (permanent kidney) develops at about five weeks in the pelvic region. It forms excretory units (nephrons) from the metanephric mesoderm and the collecting system is formed from the ureteric bud which is an outgrowth of the mesonephric duct. The metanephric tissue forms a cap over the ureteric bud and

on growth and dilatation of the bud it forms the renal pelvis, ureters, and the collecting ducts. The connection between the collecting system and the nephrons is essential for the normal development of the urinary tract. Any failure in the process will cause unilateral or bilateral renal agenesis or cystic disease (see Chapter 9). If the ureteric bud divides too early the result is bifid kidneys (duplex ureters), occasionally with ectopic ureters.

4. Answer (see Chapters 9 and 10 for a full explanation) should include two of the following:
(a) Double and bifid ureters.
(b) Uteropelvic obstruction.
(c) Ureteral or bladder diverticula.
(d) Hydroureters.
(e) Bladder extrophy.
(f) Urethral valves.
(g) Horseshoe kidney.
(h) Pelvic kidney.

5. The composition of the ultrafiltrate of plasma is dependent upon the three layers of the filtration barrier: The characteristics and functions of these three layers listed below need to be discussed (see section on the glomerulus in Chapter 2):
(a) The endothelial cells of the capillary.
(b) The basement membrane.
(c) The epithelial cells of Bowman's capsule.

6. Answer to include with examples:
(a) Diffusion.
(b) Facilatated diffusion.
(c) Primary active transport.
(d) Seconday active transport.

7. Answer (see Chapter 3) to include the use of
(a) Creatinine.
(b) Inulin.
(c) p-aminohippuric acid (PAH).
(d) Inert gas washout technique.
(e) Isotope uptake technique.
(f) ^{31}Cr EDTA.

8. (a) 10th week gestation—filtration of fluid and urine production.
(b) Newborn RBF is 5% of cardiac output—increases progressively during the first year.
(c) Postpartum GFR is 25 ml/min/1.73 m^2 body surface area.
(d) One month old—progressive increase in GFR.
(e) By one year GFR is adult value—125 ml/min.
(f) Adult RBF is 20% of cardiac output.
(g) Old age—GFR decreases progressively. Draw the graph (Fig. 3.5) to help explain.

9. Plasma glucose normal range is 2.5–5.5 mmol. About 0.2–0.5 mmol of glucose is filtered every minute with a normal plasma concentration. Any increase in the plasma glucose concentration results in a proportional increase in the amount of glucose filtered. Virtually all the filtered glucose is reabsorbed in the proximal tubule unless the filtered glucose exceeds the resorptive capacity of the cells.

(a) Glucose is transported into the proximal tubular cells against its concentration gradient by active transport (a symport). Glucose reabsorbtion is driven by energy released from the transport of sodium down its electrochemical gradient as the Na^+/K^+ ATPase pump on the basolateral membrane maintains a low sodium concentration and negative potential within the cell. Fig. 2.21 shows glucose transport in cells of the pars convoluta. The transport ratio is 1:1 sodium:glucose in the pars convoluta and 2:1 sodium:glucose in the pars recta.

(b) All the nephrons have different thresholds for glucose reabsorption (nephron heterogeneity). T_m is the maximum tubular resorptive capacity for a solute (i.e. the point of saturation for the carriers) and this value can be calculated for glucose. There is a limited number of Na^+/glucose carrier molecules and so glucose reabsorbtion is T_m limited. Fig. 2.22 shows the relationship between glucose reabsorption and excretion depending upon the plasma concentration. The graph shows that the lowest renal threshold of glucose is at a plasma glucose of 10 mmol/L. At this level filtered glucose will begin to be excreted in the urine (glycosuria). As plasma glucose concentration increases further (as may occur in uncontrolled diabetes mellitus) even the nephrons with highest resorptive capacity will allow glucose excretion and urinary glucose increases in parallel with plasma glucose. The T_m is reached at a plasma glucose concentration of 20 mmol/L.

(c) In pregnancy the renal threshold for glucose is temporarily decreased and glucose may appear in the urine even when blood glucose is less than 10 mmol/L (renal glycosuria).

10. Plasma concentration of bicarbonate is 20–30 mmol/L. Bicarbonate ions (HCO_3^-) are vital in the maintenance of acid–base balance within the body. The kidney plays an important part in the regulation of pH by controlling the plasma HCO_3^- concentration. 90% of the filtered HCO_3^- is reabsorbed into the proximal tubule and the remaining 10% is taken up in the distal tubule and collecting ducts. The reabsorption of HCO_3^- is also coupled to Na^+ transport. Fig. 2.23 illustrates the reabsorption of HCO_3^- in the proximal tubule cells.

(a) Mechanism of HCO_3^- reabsorption is as follows: Na^+ reabsorption on the apical membrane drives H^+ secretion into the tubular cells and these combine with HCO_3^- to form carbonic acid (H_2CO_3). The presence of carbonic anhydrase, on the brush border of the cells catalyses the dissociation of H_2CO_3 into H_2O and CO_2 within the tubular lumen. Both H_2O and CO_2 diffuse freely into the cell where they are recombined to form H_2CO_3 catalysed by intracellular carbonic anhydrase. HCO_3^- and Na^+ are transported out of the cell across the basolateral membrane. H^+ is secreted out of the cell into the tubular lumen and recycled to allow continuation of this cycle.

11. See Fig. 2.4.

12. Nodular and diffuse glomerulosclerosis, arteriolar lesions, and exudative lesions such as the fibrin cap are all renal manifestations of diabetes mellitus.

(a) On electron microscopy there is an increase in the thickness of the glomerular basement membrane and an increase in mesangial matrix with two morphological patterns: nodular glomerulosclerosis (Kimmelstiel–Wilson nodules)—nodular accumulations of mesangial matrix material; diffuse glomerulosclerosis—diffusely increased areas of mesangial matrix.

(b) The onset of diabetic nephropathy is clinically manifest by the development of microalbuminuria followed by overt proteinuria, which may reach the nephrotic range. There is then a progressive fall in GFR, which is commonly associated with hypertension. Diabetic nephropathy is usually associated with diabetic complications in other organs (especially retinopathy). Diabetes mellitus has usually been present for approximately 20 years before the development of end-stage renal failure. The commonest cause of needing dialysis in developed countries is chronic renal failure due to diabetes mellitus.

(c) Pyelonephritis is a common complication in patients with diabetes mellitus and can cause renal papillary necrosis.

13. (a) ACE inhibitors block ACE, which hydrolyses angiotensin I to angiotensin II. Angiotensin I is inactive and is converted in the lung to angiotensin II; this in turn is converted to angiotensin III in the adrenal gland. Angiotensin II is a very potent vasoconstrictor and aids sodium reabsorption in the tubule. The stimulus for activation of the renin–angiotensin–aldosterone system is reduced renal arteriolar pressure, sympathetic stimulation, and a reduction in the delivery of Na^+ concentration to the distal tubule.

(b) Any condition resulting in high circulating levels of renin will result in angiotensin-mediated high vascular resistance contributing to hypertension. ACE inhibitors (e.g. captopril, enalapril) inhibit the enzyme peptidyl dipeptidase, which converts angiotensin I to II and therefore lower blood pressure by decreasing peripheral vascular resistance (TPR). ACE inhibitors may also decrease blood pressure by inhibiting the local (tissue) renin–angiotensin system. ACE inhibitors have been shown to decrease proteinuria and delay the progress of renal disease in people with diabetes mellitus. They are also increasingly being used in the treatment of congestive cardiac failure.

(c) Fig. 4.5 shows the effects of ACE inhibitors.

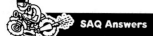

14. (a) In 2–5% of patients with hypertension the hypertension is secondary to RAS in one or both renal arteries. The stenoses may be due to fibromuscular dysplasia or atheromatous plaques (70%) within the renal artery wall. The result is excessive renin secretion by the affected kidney since there is renal hypoperfusion and this is interpreted as a fall in body fluid volume. There is also a small degree of renal ischaemia. Treatment to dilate the stenosis (angioplasty) or corrective surgery may aid blood pressure control and preserve renal function. If the blood pressure is left uncontrolled the contralateral kidney may become damaged by hypertension.

(b) People with RAS rely on constriction of the efferent renal arteriole to maintain pressures for glomerular filtration on the affected side. Angiotensin II is the main agent responsible for constriction of these vessels. On ACE inhibitor administration, a decrease in angiotensin II will dramatically decrease glomerular capillary pressure within the kidney resulting in acute renal failure.

15. (a) The ureters enter the base of the bladder at the upper border of the trigone. The bladder is a highly distensible organ. When empty, it lies in the pelvis and rests on the symphysis pubis and floor of the pelvis. When filled, it enlarges into the abdominal cavity. Partially covered by peritoneum, it has smooth muscular walls and is lined by transitional epithelium or urothelium. The neck of the bladder is relatively immobile and fixed by the puboprostatic and lateral vesical ligament (see Figs 5.4 and 5.5).

(b) The interior of the bladder is shown in Fig. 5.4. The wall is yellow with rugae (many folds) enabling greater expansion with little increase in internal pressure. The base is the trigone, a triangular reddish region. This is less mobile and does not wrinkle as the bladder contracts. It is more sensitive to painful stimuli. The bladder is lined by smooth muscle, which like the ureter is arranged in spiral, long, and circular bundles— known as the detrusor muscle.

(c) Muscle bundles surround either side of the urethra and form the internal urethral sphincter. Slightly further along the urethra, there is a skeletal muscle sphincter— the external urethral sphincter.

(d) Blood supply—the bladder is supplied by superior and inferior vesical branches of the internal iliac artery.

(e) The bladder is drained by the vesical plexus (and prostatic venous plexus in the male), which then drains into the internal iliac vein.

(f) Innervation—the bladder receives both sensory and motor parasympathetic and sympathetic innervation. The sensory innervation gives sensation (awareness) of full bladder and also pain from disease. If the bladder is empty, the impulses are suppressed. The motor parasympathetic innervation causes detrusor muscle stimulation, but inhibits the sphincter vesicae. The sympathetic innervation is inhibitory to the detrusor muscle and motor to the sphincter vesicae (see Fig. 5.7).

16. (a) 90% of the adult renal malignant tumours are RCCs. These are adenocarcinomas that arise from the tubular epithelium. RCC is very rare in children and has a peak incidence in 60–70 year olds. The male to female ratio is 3:1. It has great geographical variance with the highest incidence in Scandinavia and the lowest in South America and Africa.

(b) The predisposing factors are:

(i) Acquired cystic disease in patients who require renal replacement therapy.

(ii) von Hippel–Lindau disease.

(iii) Smoking.

(c) The tumour presents as haematuria (in 90% of cases). Non-specific symptoms include fatigue, weight loss, and fever. There may be a mass in the loin. These are all late manifestations, presenting at an advanced stage of tumour progression. 10% are clinically silent and present as metastatic disease (occult primary).

(d) Diagnosis is made by intravenous urography (IVU) and computerized tomography (CT) (see Chapter 8).

(e) A small number of RCCs secrete hormone-like substances. These hormone-like substances include:

(i) Parathyroid hormone (PTH).

(ii) Adrenocorticotrophic hormone (ACTH).

(iii) Erythropoietin.

(iv) Renin.

(f) The tumour consists of a yellow-brown well-demarcated mass in the cortex with a diameter of 3–15 cm. Within this area there are patches of haemorrhage, necrosis, and cyst formation. They are most common at the upper pole of the kidney. The renal capsule is often intact. Spread into the renal vein is often visible and rarely this extends into to the inferior vena cava. Metastases are found in the lung, liver, bone, opposite kidney, and adrenals. The TNM system is used in staging renal adenocarcinomas:

(i) T_1—confined to the kidney.

(ii) T_2—enlarging tumour with distortion of the kidney with renal capsule intact.

(iii) T_3—spread through the renal capsule into the perinephric fat with invasion into the renal vein.

(iv) T_4—invasion into adjacent organs or the abdominal wall.

(v) N—lymph node spread.

(vi) M—metastatic spread.

(g) Treatment of choice if there are no distant metastases is a radical nephrectomy. The prognosis of RCC is unpredictable and is generally determined by the degree of the spread. The average five-year survival rate is 45% and if there is no metastatic disease on presentation it increases to 70%.

17. (a) Any obstruction in the urinary tract predisposes to urinary tract infection and stone formation. Obstruction in the urinary tract can be unilateral or bilateral, complete or incomplete, gradual or sudden in onset, and if the blockage is unrelieved there is permanent renal atrophy.

(b) Careful imaging of the renal tract is essential to determine the site and cause of obstruction (see Chapter 8):

(c)   The causes of urinary obstruction are congenital abnormalities, tumours, calculi, pregnancy, hyperplastic lesions, inflammation, and neurogenic disorders.

(d)   Fig. 10.3 shows the sites of obstruction in the urinary tract.

(e)   Presentation depends upon the site and timing of the obstruction:

(i)   An acute, sudden, and complete obstruction in the ureters (e.g.a stone) will cause renal colic, which is excruciatingly painful. If unilateral, renal failure will not result.

(ii)   An insidious urethral obstruction such as a tumour in the bladder or prostatic hypertrophy will present with bladder distension and related symptoms including hesitancy, terminal dribbling, poor urine flow, and a sense of incomplete emptying. Chronic renal failure may develop.

(iii)   A unilateral and partial obstruction causing a hydroureter or hydronephrosis may not be apparent for many years since renal function is maintained by the unaffected kidney.

(iv)   A bilateral and partial obstruction presents with nocturia and polyuria due to tubular cell dysfunction and therefore diminished ability to concentrate urine. Other manifestations include salt wasting, distal tubular acidosis, hypertension, and chronic renal failure.

(v)   A bilateral and complete obstruction presents as anuria or oliguria with acute renal failure. It is not compatible with life without release of the blockage. On release there is a massive postobstructive diuresis that leaves the patient susceptible to dehydration.

(vi)   General malaise or fever may be a sign that infection is complicating the obstruction.

(f)   Hydronephrosis is the dilatation of the renal pelvis and calyces that is associated with any obstruction in the urinary tract. This will go on to produce progressive atrophy of the kidney since the backpressure of the obstruction is transmitted into the distal parts of the nephron and the GFR progressively declines. Progressive damage to the renal structures causes flattening of the calyces with gradual thinning of the renal parenchyma and can lead to a complete loss of normal architecture, leaving behind a cystic, thin-walled fibrous sac with no functional capacity.

18. (a)   The anion gap represents the difference between the concentration of the major plasma cations (Na^+) and the major plasma anions (Cl^- and HCO_3^-). Calculations of the anion gap provide a convenient way for analysing and help in determining the cause of a metabolic acidosis.

(b)   Indications for measuring the anion gap are confusion, lethargy, seizures, coma, arrhythmia, hypertension, hypotension, vomiting, diarrhoea, heavy sweating, diabetes mellitus, polyuria, polydypsia.

(c)   Anion gap = $([K^+]+[Na^+]) - ([Cl^-] - [HCO_3^-])$
 Normal anion gap = $8-16\,mmol/L$

(d)   Increased anion gap is found in renal failure lacticacidosis (from shock), anion ingestion (salicylate poisioning), ketoacidosis (diabetes mellitus). The metabolic acidosis resulting from diarrhoea and renal tubular acidosis is associated with a normal anion gap.

19. (a) In-situ immune complex deposition. Immune complexes are formed within the kidney. The antibodies react with intrinsic or planted antigens within the glomerulus. Anti-glomerular basement membrane (GBM) disease is an example involving intrinsic antigen. Antibodies are formed against an antigen in the GBM. The complex elicits the complement cascade, leading to severe damage to the glomerulus and rapidly progressing renal failure. The anti-GBM antibodies also attack the basement membrane of the alveoli in the lungs. The association of anti-GBM antibodies, glomerulonephritis (GN), and pulmonary haemorrhage is known as Goodpasture's syndrome. Planted antigens are antigens planted within the glomerulus and not of renal origin. They can be:

(i)   Exogenous—for example bacteria such as group A β-haemolytic streptococcus. This results in post-streptococcal GN. Other antigens include bacterial products (endostreptosin), aggregated IgG, viruses, parasites, and drugs.

(ii)   Endogenous—for example nucleic acid—antibodies react with host DNA as seen in systemic lupus erythematosus (SLE).

(b)   Circulating immune complex nephritis. Here, immune complexes are not formed within the kidney. They are formed elsewhere and get trapped within the glomerulus from the renal circulation. When trapped in the glomerulus the immune complex causes an inflammatory reaction resulting in damage to the glomerulus. On immunofluorescence microscopy, granular deposits are seen along the basement membrane and/or in the mesangium. Once again the antigen may be:

(i)   Exogenous—for example bacteria (group A streptococci, *Treponema pallidum*), surface antigen of hepatitis B, hepatitis C virus antigen, tumour antigens, viruses.

(ii)   Endogenous—DNA in SLE.

(c)   Cytotoxic antibodies. Antibodies to glomerular cell antigens are formed and cause damage without any deposits—for example antibodies fixing to mesangial cells and causing complement-mediated mesangiolysis and mesangial cell proliferation. Experimental examples of this are known in rats, but it is not clear that this occurs in man.

(d)   Cell-mediated immunity. Sensitized T cells from cell-mediated immune reactions may cause glomerular injury. This form of damage is important in progressive GN. It is thought that macrophages and T lymphocytes are present and mediate damage in the glomerulus in such cases.

(e)   Activation of the alternative complement pathway. Bacterial polysaccharides, endotoxins, and IgA aggregates may activate the alternative complement pathway and give rise to components that then deposit

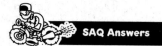

in the glomeruli causing damage. This mechanism is seen in membranoproliferative GN.

20. The complications of prolonged obstruction of urine flow are associated with compensatory hypertrophy of the bladder wall as a result of high pressure that develops within the bladder (Fig. 10.8) and are as follows:
(a) Bands of thickened smooth muscle fibre cause trabeculation of the bladder wall.
(b) Diverticula formation on the external surface of the bladder.
(c) Bladder dilation once the muscle becomes hypotonic.
(d) Hydroureter formation resulting in reflux of urine up to the renal pelvis.
(e) Bilateral hydronephrosis.
(e) Kidney infection, stones, and renal failure.

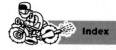

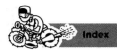

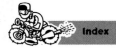

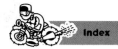

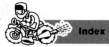

renal infarction, 148
renal insufficiency, 146
renal mass, 135, 149
renal medulla, 13
   hypertonicity, 33–6
renal osteodystrophy, 73, 112, 114
renal pelvis, 15, 75
   stones, 154
renal plasma flow, 40
renal replacement therapy, 73–4
renal stones *see* renal calculi
renal transplantation, 74, 127, 128
   malakoplakia vesicae in, 156
renal tubules, 3, 14
   atrophy, 141
   diseases, 28, 142–6
   injury, 142
   organization, 15
   sodium transport, 25–6
   transport processes in, 23–6
   see also distal tubule; proximal tubule
renin, 16, 48
   release, 16, 48, 50
   release in renal artery stenosis, 66
   tumours producing, 149
renin–angiotensin–aldosterone system, 48–9
   stimulation in liver disease, 67
renography, DTPA, 153
respiratory acidosis, 54, 55
   causes, 55
respiratory alkalosis, 54, 56
   causes, 56
respiratory signs, renal disease, 111
respiratory system, examination, 113
retinal changes, 110
retinal–renal syndromes, 135
retrograde pyelography, 121, 127, 153
retroperitoneal fibrosis, 90, 126
rubidium, 40

S

Schistosoma, 155
Schistosoma haematobium, 156
schistosomiasis, 126, 155, 156
scleral deposits, 110
secondary active transport, 25
secretion, 23, 30
   gradient time-limited mechanisms, 31
   T_m-limited mechanisms, 30–1
seminal fluid, 79
septicaemia, 143, 144
serological tests, 91
sexually transmitted diseases, 157, 160

shifting dullness, 118
shock, 64, 142
single injection method, 9
skin colour, signs of renal disease, 109, 110
slit pores, 19
smoking, 149, 157
social history, 86
sodium (Na+), 6, 25–6
   aldosterone effect, 37, 49
   angiotensin II action, 48
   balance, 48
   composition of fluid compartments, 8
   control of aldosterone release, 49
   control of effective circulating volume, 48
   diffusion, 7, 25
   entry into proximal tubule cells, 26–7
   extrusion into lateral space, 26
   normal values, 95, 123
   reabsorption, 24, 25, 32, 49–50
   reabsorption reduced by CA inhibitors, 70
   reabsorption reduced by diuretics, 69
   retention, 67
   solute transport associated, 27, 27–30
   transport in loop of Henle, 26, 32, 33
   transport processes/mechanisms, 7, 24, 25, 26
   transport in proximal tubule, 26, 26–7
   see also hypernatraemia; hyponatraemia
sodium pump *see* Na+/K+ ATPase
solutes
   osmoreceptor sensitivity to changes, 44
   output, effect on urine volume, 47
   transport in proximal tubule, 27, 27–30
solvents, organic, 142
sphincter insufficiency, 102
spinal cord lesions, 81, 153
spinal shock, 81
spironolactone, 68, 69
squamous cell carcinoma, 158–9
squamous metaplasia, 157, 158
staghorn calculi, 125, 154
Staphylococcus, 143, 160
Starling forces, 21, 22, 49
stature, 109
sterile cystitis, 155
stones
   kidney *see* renal calculi
   urinary tract, 154–5
streptococcal antigen, 122
streptococci, group A β-haemolytic, 68, 138
stress incontinence, 102
sulphate, transport in proximal tubule, 30
superior frontal gyrus, lesions, 80
suppurative cystitis, 155

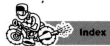